YOGA
FOR BEGINNERS

Your Guide To Conscious Meditation, Sattvic Diet And Postures For Weight Loss, Stress Reduction and Personal Well-Being

Jane Kundal Meditation Class

© **Copyright 2020 Jane Kundall Meidtation Class**

All rights reserved

This document is geared towards providing exact and reliable information with regards to the topic and issue covered. The publication is sold with the idea that the publisher is not required to render accounting, officially permitted, or otherwise, qualified services. If advice is necessary, legal or professional, a practiced individual in the profession should be ordered.

From a Declaration of Principles which was accepted and approved equally by a Committee of the American Bar Association and a Committee of Publishers and Associations.

In no way is it legal to reproduce, duplicate, or transmit any part of this document in either electronic means or in printed format. Recording of this publication is strictly prohibited and any storage of this document is not allowed unless with written permission from the publisher. All rights reserved

The information provided herein is stated to be truthful and consistent, in that any liability, in terms of inattention or otherwise, by any usage or abuse of any policies, processes, or directions contained within is the solitary and utter responsibility of the recipient reader. Under no circumstances will any legal responsibility or blame be held against the publisher for any reparation, damages, or monetary loss due to the information herein, either directly or indirectly.

Respective authors own all copyrights not held by the publisher.

The information herein is offered for informational purposes solely and is universal as so. The presentation of the information is without contract or any type of guarantee assurance.

The trademarks that are used are without any consent, and the publication of the trademark is without permission or backing by the trademark owner. All trademarks and brands within this book are for clarifying purposes only and are the owned by the owners themselves, not affiliated with this document.

INTRODUCTION	7
HISTORY OF YOGA- MAJOR HISTORICAL TIME FRAMES	9
Vedic period (circa 1500–600 BCE)	9
Modern era	11
FOUNDATIONS OF YOGA PRACTICE	13
THE EIGHT LIMBS OF YOGA	15
YOGA TERMINOLOGIES	21
A DEEP UNDERSTANDING OF YOGA	31
Yoga as a science	32
DEVICES AND INNOVATION OF (YOGA VIDHI)	34
THE TRUE PURPOSE OF YOGA	36
True Yoga: Beyond the Body	38
THIS IS THE GENUINE MOTIVATION BEHIND YOGA.	40
PRE-YOGA ORIENTATION AND PREPARATION	56
Before You Start	56
THE MOST EFFECTIVE METHOD TO PRACTICE	60
BASIC YOGA POSES	67
Sun Salutations	68
Sitting Poses	83
Knees Poses	93
Closing Poses & Mudras	97
BASIC YOGA ROUTINES	99
Sun Salutations	100

One hand backbend	105
Revolved triangle pose	106
Wide leg forward bend I	110
Wide leg forward twist	111
Warrior pose I	112
Warrior pose II	113
Simple warrior present III	114
Easy half moon pose	115
Standing Half Bow Balance	118
Standing Knee To Chest Balance	119
Falcon Pose	121
Pussyfoot Pose	124
Simple Meditation Pose	125
Half Lotus Pose	126
Lotus Pose	128
Jolt Pose I	129
Two Legs Forward Bend I	130
Two Legs Forward Bend II	131
Contorted Pose I	132
Twisted Pose II	134
Sitting Half Boat Pose	135
Twisted Forward Stretch	136
Hip Rocking Pose	137
Butterfly Pose	138

Shoemaker's Pose 140

Knees Poses 141

Cat Stretch 142

Alternate Leg-Hand Balance 143

Tiger Pose 144

Downward Facing Dog 145

Raised Leg Downward Facing Dog 146

Closing Poses & Mudras 147

Surya Mudra 148

Mountain Pose 150

Side Mountain Pose 151

Surrender Pose 152

YOGA DIET 155

TABLE SHOWING SATTVIC, RAJASIC AND TAMASIC ARTICLES OF DIET 171

FREQUENTLY ASKED QUESTIONS 173

    Do you need rest days from yoga? 174

    What do I need to begin yoga? 175

    Imagine a scenario in which I nod off or wheeze during Savasana. 177

    Five Easy Mindfulness Meditations 179

REPRESENTATIONS 184

BRAINWAVE ENTRAINMENT 186

SIXTEEN PRINCIPLES OF SELF DEFENSE 188

LADIES, YOGA, AND SELF-DEFENSE: HOW THE SPECKS ASSOCIATE.. 191

SURVIVAL FITNESS PLAN YOGA ROUTINE QUICK-LIST 199

METHODS AND DRILLS TO IMPROVE YOUR SWIMMING VELOCITY... 202

    How to do the Survival Fitness Plan Super Burpee. A warm-up, stretch, and conditioning workout all in one exercise 203

CONCLUSION 208

INTRODUCTION

Yoga is not just a process but also a goal. In this respect, it is a moksha Shastra, teaching (Shastra), leading to gradual freedom (moksha) from the various forms of human suffering. The word yoga is derived from the Sanskrit verb root YUJ, which means **"to yoke, unite, or bring together."** Yoga may be defined as the effort to restore harmony within the body-mind complex and as the effort to reunite the individual human spirit with its essential nature. Although the practice of yoga does not exclude any religion, creed, or race, it is helpful to recognize that its teachings have sprung from the spiritual soil of ancient India and even now bear the title in India of Sanatana dharma, "eternal way." Although yoga has been practiced in India since well before recorded history, it was in approximately the second century BCE that the seminal figure Patanjali united many already-existing practices and writings into a unified text known as the Yoga Sutras.

Patanjali's masterful Sanskrit work contains a series of 195 brief aphorisms (sutras, or "threads") that convey essential ideas of yoga theory and practice. These sutras present the essence of yoga in the form of eight divisions, or limbs (ashtanga yoga). The first five limbs of this system are termed "external" because they address relationships with the world and with the body, breath, and senses. The "internal," or "mental," rungs of yoga, the last three of the eight limbs, comprise three increasingly refined stages of concentration. At the heart of the text of Patanjali is the message that every human being is healthy and whole by nature. Yoga is a way to align yourself with a sense of inner harmony. In the process, multiple levels of human experience—body, breath, and mind—are given thorough attention, and the mind is gradually freed for deeper concentration and reflection. Many modern practitioners have become interested in yoga as a means of improving health. Patanjali recognized imbalances in health as a significant obstacle to personal progress and approached the task of promoting good health in two ways: by removing barriers that block the path to health and by developing alignment with healing forces within. As we shall see, these two strategies are manifested in a wide variety of approaches to self-management. It is essential to recognize that the modern, almost exclusive, identification of yoga with physical exercise is just that—a recent development. As Patanjali illustrates, yoga practices in earlier times embodied a thoroughly integrated approach. They combined in one system the goals of improved health, self-discovery, and spiritual self-understanding.

HISTORY OF YOGA- MAJOR HISTORICAL TIME FRAMES

Vedic period (circa 1500–600 BCE)

In the period before written texts, teachings were transmitted orally from the teacher (guru) to disciple (shishya). The earliest of these teachings are found today in four compilations: the Rig Veda, the Yajur Veda, the Sama Veda, and the Atharva Veda. The age of these works has been a matter of some uncertainty. It is estimated that although the oral tradition extends far back into prehistory, the Vedas as they are organized today, date from circa 1500 BCE, with later additions extending to 600 BCE. Each Veda (from the root vid, "to know") consists of four parts. The Samhitas, collections of hymns used in Vedic rituals, form the oldest portion. The Brahmanas and Aranyakas comment on and expand the Samhitas, while the Upanishads form the final part of the texts. The Vedas promote harmonious relationships with nature, appeal for peace in human interactions, petition for health and protection, and, most importantly, bring awareness to the meditative dimensions of human life. Post-Vedic era (circa 600 to 100 BCE).

In the period following the compilation of the Vedas, an enormous collection of teachings was recorded and made available for practice and study. Twelve Upanishads and their comprehensive interpretation, the Brahma Sutras, began the shift away from Vedic rituals to the highly personalized yogic goals of self- development, balanced living, and Self-realization. Diverse literature emerged that included two epic texts, the Ramayana and Mahabharata, and the latter's famous quintessence, the Bhagavad Gita. Yoga practices were codified in the Yoga Sutras of Patanjali (c. 200–100 BCE), and Patanjali's writing was accompanied by an authoritative commentary added by the sage Vyasa.

One hundred BCE and through the seventeenth century CE During the common era, devotional works, histories, and teachings of yogic adepts all provided a resource for practicing yogis. The renowned philosopher Shankaracharya (eighth century CE) had a profound influence on the thought of this period. He revived the doctrine of Advaita Vedanta, nondualism, and wrote authoritative commentaries on the Bhagavad Gita, the Brahma Sutras, and ten principal Upanishads. During this period, many types of yoga emerged from within the diverse traditions of India. Georg Feuerstein (2003) has listed 40 types of yoga, ranging across a broad array of practice approaches. Among these, the three main ones surviving into the modern age are the Yoga Sutras of Patanjali; the hatha yoga teachings of the Natha sect of yogis (in particular, a fifteenth-century work by Svatmarama, the Hatha Yoga Pradipika, and a seventeenth-century work of Gheranda, the Gheranda Samhita); and the teachings of the Bhagavad Gita.

Modern era

In the modern period, yoga and its teachings traveled from East to West; a phenomenon embodied first by the arrival of Swami Vivekananda in the United States in 1893. Drawing on the teachings of the Bhagavad Gita, he wrote on each of the four paths found there: raja yoga (meditation), karma yoga (selfless action), bhakti yoga (devotion), and jnana yoga (metaphysics). In the early twentieth century, Swami Kuvalayananda of the Kaivalyadhama Yoga Institute, as well as Yogendraji of the Yoga Institute in Mumbai, initiated systematic practice and research in yoga. Since then, various traditions have spread worldwide. These include teachings set in motion by T. Krishnamacharya (who inspired well-known practitioners of yoga such as B. K. S. Iyengar, T. K. V. Desikachar, and Pattabhi Jois); Swami Shivananda Sarasvati (and his disciples Swamis Satyananda, Vishnudevananda, and Satchitananda); the Himalayan tradition (Swami Rama, Pandit Tigunait, and Swami Veda Bharati); the Kundalini Yoga tradition (Yogi Bhajan); the Self-Realization Fellowship

(Swami Yogananda); and the Rishiculture of Swami Gitananda Giri (Yogacharini Meenakshi Devi Bhavanani). Yoga practitioners and scientists such as H. R. Nagendra and R. Nagarathna of S-VYASA (Swami Vivekananda Yoga Anusandhana Samsthana) University in Bangalore continued the early efforts of Swami Kuvalayananda with a particular emphasis on yoga as therapy. Since 2002, Swami Ramdev has popularized yoga throughout India as well as initiating research to study its effectiveness in health care. Other recent schools of practice are listed in the final part of this chapter. Notably, while yoga teachings have been derived from many written sources, it is the presence of a living lineage of teachers (a guruparampara) that assures that a particular teaching is genuine.

FOUNDATIONS OF YOGA PRACTICE

In the initial stages of yoga study, most students focus on postures (asana), voluntary regulation of the breath (pranayama), and relaxation skills (pratyahara). Integrated with contemplation of the yamas and niyamas (described below), these form the foundation for the development of effective practice. However, it is helpful to broaden the focus here to provide a philosophical context and illustrate how yoga techniques expand into daily life. Yoga is indeed a way of life and experiential investigation into human nature. (See Table 1) The essence of yoga is self-observation. It is through self-observation, for example, that the refinement of yoga postures occurs. In the course of asana work, self-observation brings with it a sense of psychological distance from the body—a perception that there is space between the witnessing mind and the movements and alignment of the physical self. A unique sense of objectivity develops—an awareness that the observer, the process of observation (carried out in mind), and the object being observed (the body and its movements) are distinct parts of an integrated inner experience, this, in turn, leads to a deep sense of physical self-mastery and the feeling that one's body has become "like the wide expanse of the sky" (Ananta samapatti).

Table 1 The eight limbs of Yoga

Table 1 The eight limbs of Yoga	
Ashtanga Yoga— the eight limbs	

1 **Yama**
  Ahimsa
  Satya
  Asteya
  Brahmacharya
  Aparigraha
	Restraints
	Non-harming
	Truthfulness
	Non-stealing
	Control of lifestyle
	Non-possessiveness

2 **Niyama**
  Shaucha
  Santosha
  Tapas
  Svadhyaya
  Ishvara pranidhana
	Observances
	Purity
	Contentment
	Self-discipline
	Self-study
	Trustful surrender

3 **Asana** 4 **Pranayama** 5 **Pratyahara** 6 **Dharana** 7 **Dhyana** 8 **Samadhi**	Steady posture Expansion of vital energy Sensory withdrawal Concentration Meditation Self-realization

A similar but more subtle process occurs when the breath becomes the object of attention. In this regard, it is often declared that without the breath, there is no yoga. Observation of the breath calms emotional reactivity, heightens awareness of the energetic dimensions of human life, and awakens the witnessing mind. Breath awareness begins with continuous awareness of the flow of exhalation and inhalation. Each exhalation provides a pleasant sensation of cleansing. At the same time, each inhalation offers an equally satisfying sense of nourishment—attention to these streams of air results in the development of effortless, relaxed breathing. The most refined event of self- observation occurs in meditation. There, the process of witnessing lies entirely within the mind itself. The ever-present stream of thought, emotions, memories, sensations, and states of consciousness forms an object of attention. Gradually, when the attention steadies the awareness of the mind, the individual's identity when the inner witness is exposed and consciousness rest within itself.

THE EIGHT LIMBS OF YOGA

The ashtanga ("eight-limbed") yoga system of Patanjali, as described in the Yoga Sutras, provides the discipline, guidance, and vision necessary for an understanding of yoga. Although the first five limbs form steps leading to meditation, practitioners are not expected to perfect these before proceeding on. Learning yoga is an organic process, and the various practices of yoga mutually clarify and support one another until the higher limbs can be achieved. The first two limbs of training consist of strategies devoted to self-regulation. They begin with the yamas, or "restraints," a list of five approaches (see Table 2) for controlling negative habit patterns that distributed energy in the individual and foster human discord. The Yamas offer a concise approach to self-inspection. By identifying negative tendencies and fostering positive ones, practitioners can recognize underlying motivations that disrupt behavior. Thus, while at one level these restraints supply a set of ethical disciplines for practice, at a deeper level, they are a tool for self-understanding, enabling practitioners to recognize the excessive attractions and aversions that so quickly become ingrained in daily life. The second rung of the ashtanga system is a list of observances (niyamas)—positive habit patterns that guide yoga practice. These principles form a framework that can be embraced at beginning levels as well as more advanced ones. For example, beginning students learn such techniques as nasal irrigation. Advancing students address the purification of the mind. The practices associated with the five observances are multi-dimensional. Svadhyaya (self-study), for example, includes not only efforts to practice introspection but also the repetition of mantras, contemplation of philosophical ideals, and attention to teachings of accomplished teachers.

The remaining six rungs in the ashtanga system are composed of increasingly refined disciplines leading toward inner stillness. Patanjali famously defines the culmination of asana work as a posture that has become "steady and comfortable." Breathing reaches its apex when it becomes a means for revealing inner awareness. And the senses, paradoxically, become a source of insight when they can be turned away from their objects and rested. Each of these stages of practice is itself a goal of yoga—each contributing to the awakening of a state of consciousness that transcends ordinary awareness. The processes of yoga culminate in freedom from the wandering tendencies of the mind; This is achieved through the implementation of two interwoven practices: concentration and non-attachment. Together these lead an aspirant to self-mastery.

Patanjali teaches that concentration practice bears fruit when it is continued over time and without interruption. But concentration is not, in this context, the result of labored attention. It is the outcome of resting awareness in a supportive focus, an alambana and returning to that focus with regularity. With modest effort, periods of concentration become a natural part of daily life. The companion to strength, vairagya, or non-attachment, is a concept that has proved puzzling for Western students. In the West, attachment is generally considered to be a desirable thing, an indication of love and respect. These virtues, love, and respect, are equally valued in yoga. But in yoga, the term "attachment" is unrelated to qualities of endearment. Attachment is seen as an imbalance, a craving leading to sickness or to mental distraction.

Non-attachment is its opposite, a sense of serenity and emotional balance. The highest state of meditation, and the eighth rung of the ashtanga system, is termed samadhi. It is described as a state of mental purity arising from one-pointed attention. In that state, consciousness is revealed as something more than a quality of mind. Mindfulness is the nature of one's being.

	Table 2
Forms of yoga	
Ashtanga yoga	The eight-limbed system outlined by Patanjali and forming the basis for all classic approaches to Yoga practice
Hatha yoga	The initial stages of ashtanga yoga practice emphasizing right attitudes, asana, breathwork, and relaxation
Raja yoga	The meditative stages of ashtanga yoga leading from

	resting the senses to deep states of relaxation, concentration, and meditation
Karma yoga	A yogic path focusing on selflessness and non-attachment. A path that accompanies all other disciplines of practice
Bhakti yoga	A sacred path often demonstrated through chant, poetry, ritual, pilgrimage, and expressions of love for the Infinite.
Jnana yoga	A path dedicated to philosophical clarity and self-observation. This approach integrates self-analysis and meditation
Tantra yoga	A highly integrated, holistic path; the umbrella for much of the practice now taught in yoga

	classes and depicted in yoga texts
Mantra yoga	An approach emphasizing the use of internal mantric sounds for mental support and the refinement of awareness
Kundalini yoga	A path dedicated to arousing dormant spiritual energy (kundalini) and directing it upward along the spinal axis
Laya yoga	A method contributing to kundalini awakening through the systematic integration of lower energies into higher ones
Svara yoga	An advanced yoga practice dedicated to the study of pranic rhythms and internal paths of energy

YOGA TERMINOLOGIES

1. **Acarya** (in some cases spelled Acharya in English): a preceptor, teacher; master
2. **Advaita** (non-duality): reality and instructing that there is just a single reality
3. **Ahimsa** (non-hurting): the absolute most significant reasonable control (Yama)
4. **Ananda** (delight): the state of absolute bliss, which is a fundamental nature of the ultimate reality
5. **Anga** (appendage): a central class of the yogic way, for example, asana, Dharana, dhyana, niyama, pranayama, pratyahara, samadhi, yama
6. **Ardha** (half)
7. **Asana** (seat): a physical stance; the third appendage (anga) of Patanjali's eight overlap way (astha-anga-yoga); initially this implied just contemplation pose
8. **Ashrama** (that where exertion is made): seclusion; likewise a phase of life
9. **Atman** (self): the supernatural Spirit, which is everlasting and; our actual nature or identity
10. **Avidya** (numbness): the primary driver of misery

11. **Ayurveda, Ayur-veda** (life science): one of India's conventional frameworks of medication
12. **Bandha** (security/servitude): the way that individuals are usually bound by numbness which makes them lead a real existence represented by karmic propensity as opposed to the inward opportunity created through astuteness
13. **Bhagavad Gita** (Lord's Song): the most established yoga book discovered
14. **Mahabharata Bhakta** (aficionado): a devotee rehearsing bhakti yoga
15. **Bhakti** (dedication/love): the affection for the bhakta toward the Divine
16. **Bhakti** (Yoga of commitment): a significant part of the yoga convention.
17. **Bindu** (seed/point): the innovative strength of anything where all energies are engaged; the spot (likewise called tilaka) worn on the temple as demonstrative of the third eye
18. **Brahma** (Creator): the Creator of the universe
19. **Brahmacharya** (from brahma and acarya "Brahmic lead"): the order of modesty
20. **Brahman** (The Supreme Atman): a definitive Reality
21. **Brahmana or Brahmin**: an individual from the most noteworthy social class of conventional Indian culture

22. **Cakra or Chakra** (wheel): actually, the wheel of a wagon
23. **Darshana** (seeing): vision in the strict and figurative sense; an arrangement of theory.
24. **Dharana** (holding): the practice of fixation, the 6th appendage (anga) of Patanjali's eight-limbed yoga
25. **Dhyana** (ideating): reflection, the seventh appendage (anga) of Patanjali's eight-limbed yoga
26. **Dharma** (strict way)
27. **Diksha** (inception): the demonstration and state of acceptance into the shrouded parts of yoga or a specific ancestry of educators; all customary yoga is initiatory
28. **Drishti** (see/sight): yogic looking, for example, at the tip of the nose or the spot between the eyebrows
29. **Gayatri-mantra**: a well known Vedic mantra recounted especially at dawn
30. **Guna** (quality): a term that has various implications, including "uprightness."
31. **Master** (profoundly edified soul): an otherworldly instructor
32. **Master bhakti** (instructor dedication): a devotee's self-rising above commitment to the master
33. **Master Gita** (Guru's Song): a book in recognition of the master, regularly chantedin ashramas

34. **Master Yoga** (Yoga [relating to] the instructor): a yogic methodology that makes theguru the support of a supporter's training
35. **Hatha Yoga** (Forceful Yoga): a significant part of yoga, stressing the physical components of the transformative way, remarkably poses (asana) and purging methods (shodhana), yet additionally breath control (pranayama)
36. **Hatha-Yoga-Pradipika** ("Light on Hatha Yoga"): This is one of three traditional manuals on hatha yoga, written by Svatmarama Yogendra in the fourteenth century
37. **Ida-Nadi** (pale conductor): the prana current or circular segment rising on the left side of the focal channel (Sushumna Nadi) related with the parasympathetic nervous framework and having a cooling or quieting impact on the psyche when activated
38. **Ishvara** (ruler): the Lord, alluding either to the CreatorIshvara-pranidhana (commitment to the Lord): Devotion to the Lord.
39. **Japa** (talk delicately) the recitation of mantras
40. **Jiva-atman, jivatman** (singular self): the individuated awareness, as opposed to a definitive Self (parama-atman)

41. **Jnana** (data/insightfulness): both primary data or world-transcending wisdom, dependent upon the unique circumstance
42. **Jnana** (Yoga of shrewdness): the way to freedom dependent on knowledge
43. **Kaivalya** (separation): the condition of total opportunity from adapted.
44. **Kali**: a Goddess epitomizing the savage (dissolving) part of the Divine
45. **Kali-yuga**: the dim time of otherworldly and ethical decrease, said to be present now; kali doesn't allude to the Goddess Kali however to the losing toss of a bite the dust
46. **Kama** (want): the craving for erotic delight hindering the way to truebliss
47. **Kapal** (skull): cerebrumKarman
48. **Karma** (activity): movement of any sort.
49. **Karma** (Yoga of activity): the freeing way of self-rising above activity
50. **Karuna** (empathy): widespread sympathy.
51. **Kosha** (packaging): any of five "envelopes" encompassing the (atman)
52. **Kumbhaka**: breath maintenance.
53. **Kundalini**-Yoga: the yogic way concentrating on the kundalini procedure as a means of freedom
54. **Maha** (amazing)

55. **Maha bandha** (the Great lock) joins the three secures yoga – together with breath maintenance.
56. **Mahabharata** (Great Bharata): one of India's two extraordinary old sagas telling of the incredible war between the Pandavas and the Kauravas and filling in as a repository for some otherworldly and suitable lessons
57. **Mahatma** (from maha-atman, "extraordinary self"): an honorific tittle
58. **Manas** (mind): the psyche, which is bound to the faculties and yields information rather than astuteness
59. **Mandala** (circle): A round structure which symbolizes the universe and expresses it to a god
60. **Mantra** (from the linguistic root word, "to think"): A hallowed sound or expression.
61. **Mantra**-Yoga: the yogic way of using mantras as the essential methods for freedom
62. **Maya** (she who quantifies): the deceiving or illusive intensity of the world.
63. **Moksha** (discharge): the state of opportunity from obliviousness
64. **Mudra** (seal): a hand signal or entire body motion
65. **Muni** (he who is quiet): a sage

66. **Nadi** (course): one of at least 72,000 unpretentious channels along or through which the existence power (prana) circles, of which the three most significant ones are the Ida-Nadi, Pingala-Nadi, and Sushumna-Nadi

67. **Nadi-shodhana** (channel purging): the act of cleaning the conduits, especially by methods for breath control (pranayama)

68. **Nirodha** (limitation): in Patanjali's eight-limbed yoga, the very premise of the procedure of fixation, contemplation, and rapture.

69. **Mantra**-Yoga: the yogic way of using mantras as the essential methods for freedom

70. **Maya** (she who gauges): the beguiling or illusive intensity of the world.

71. **Moksha** (discharge): the state of opportunity from numbness

72. **Mudra** (seal): a hand motion or entire body signal

73. **Muni** (he who is quiet): a sage

74. **Nadi** (conductor): one of at least 72,000 inconspicuous channels along or through which the existence power (prana) circles, of which the three most significant ones are the Ida-Nadi, Pingala-Nadi, and Sushumna-Nadi

75. **Nadi-shodhana** (channel purging): the act of filtering the conduits, especially by methods for breath control (pranayama)
76. **Nirodha** (limitation): in Patanjali's eight-limbed yoga, the very premise of the procedure of focus, reflection, and joy.
77. **Niyama** ([self-]restraint): the second appendage of Patanjali's eight overlap way
78. **Ojas** (imperativeness): the inconspicuous vitality delivered through training, particularly the order of virtue (brahmacharya)
79. **Om**: the first mantra symbolizing a definitive Reality, which is prefixed to numerous mantric expressions
80. **Pada** (foot)
81. **Padmasana** (lotus represent): a situated reflective stance
82. **Parama-atman or paramatman** (incomparable self): the supernatural Self
83. **Parama-hamsa, Paramahansa** (incomparable swan): an honorific title given to incredible adepts
84. **Patanjali**: Yoga Sutra compiler who has lived c. CE 150
85. **Pingala-Nadi** (rosy conductor): the prana current or circular segment rising on the right side of

the focal channel (Sushumna-Nadi) and related to the sympathetic sensory system and energizingly affecting the brain when enacted.

86. **Prana** (life/breath): life by and large; the existence power supporting the body; the breath as an outer indication of the inconspicuous life power

87. **Pranayama** (from prana and Ayama, "life/breath expansion"): breath control, the fourth appendage (anga) of Patanjali's eight overlap way

88. **Prasada** (beauty/lucidity): divine elegance; mental clearness

89. **Pratyahara** (withdrawal): tactile restraint, the fifth appendage of Patanjali's eight overlay way

90. **Puja** (adore): custom love, which is a significant part of numerous structures of yoga.

91. **Puraka**: inward breath, a part of breath control

92. **Purana** (Ancient [History]): a sort of mainstream reference book managing royal genealogy, cosmology, theory, and custom; there are eighteen significant and many progressively minor works of this nature

93. **Sat** (being/reality/truth): the ultimate RealitySatya (truth/truthfulness): truth, a designation of the ultimate Reality; also the practice of honesty, which is an aspect of moral discipline

94. **Shakti** (power): the supreme feminine component of Reality.
95. **Shishya** (student/disciple): the initiated disciple of the Shodhana guru (cleansing/purification): an essential feature of all yogic paths; a group of purification practices in the Shraddha hatha yoga (faith): an essential disposition on the Shuddhi yogic path (purification/purity): the state of purity; a synonym for the Shodhana path
96. **Siddhi** (accomplishment/perfection): spiritual perfection, the attainment of flawless identity with the ultimate Reality (atman or brahman); paranormal ability, of which the yoga tradition knows many kinds
97. **Tapas** (heat): austerity, penance, which is an ingredient of all yogic approaches, since they all involve self-transcendence
98. **Upanishad** (sitting near): a type of scripture representing the concluding portion of the revealed literature of Hinduism

A DEEP UNDERSTANDING OF YOGA

Yoga is a true way of life; it is also an experiential science of human nature that helps us to realize our real being." Take up the study of yoga science like any other science of material existence and note that it does not contain any mystery or risk" (Vivekananda, 1896). Yoga is the original, eternal "essence" wisdom. The study of infinite human possession may adequately be called Yoga. Yoga may properly be called the science of limitless human possibilities because it allows us to manifest our intrinsic potentialities in entirety. Yoga deals concurrently with all facets of conscious evolutionary theory, psychology, and practicality. Yoga does have not only the ideas but also the requisite tools and technologies to identify and understand the "essence" Yoga helps one to reach the complexities of the being theoretically, but first of all, experientially.

Ornish and Taimini have a significant role to illustrate the significance of yoga. "Yoga is a system of ideal tools for union and healing" (Ornish, 2010), though Taimni calls yoga "science of sciences."

Yoga as a science

Yoga can be considered to be a body of wisdom transmitted from Guru to Chela over millennia. It was accomplished by intense, systematic, introverted research into the workings of the human mind in pursuit of the meaning of life. The critical theory is that the human being is, in fact, the "divine being," and therefore, entirely able for experience Sat Chit Anandam. Since the mind controls matter (the mind controls the body, thoughts, and emotions), our birthright (possibilities) is safety and happiness, so freedom from all restriction (moksha) is the objective of human existence. General laws regulating the mind, the emotions, and the body were discovered through the thousands of years of introverted study, thus finding out that living following these universal laws (Sanatana Dharma) creates harmony, health, happiness, and spiritual growth.

Yoga science can be viewed as distillation and sublimation of all the finest, noblest behaviors leftover as the legacy of the sages of yoga (rishis), a treasure trove of learning. The old Indian sacred texts Vedas and Upanishads are the home of the treasury, where these valuable perspectives are guarded for keeping. The insightful soul realizes how to manage this treasurer and utilize the abundance of information contained in that.

Yoga has the terminology used to describe various phenomena, as well as the technology in the form of excellent instruments (asanas, pranayama, kriyas, mudras, bandhas, shat karma, etc.) to unify and use this truth in daily life discover Yoga has the philosophy of an experiential and exploratory methodology which suggests execution of the different physical and mental activities (abhyasa) and watching the resultant impacts with an impartial feeling of objectivity (vairagya). Yoga additionally has an amassed assemblage of information through centuries, as the consequence of experiential and trial concentrates by the incomparable Rishis as recorded in the Vedas, Upanishads, Puranas, Itihasas, Shastras and so on. The last viewpoint, the 'reality,' is that these encounters are available to confirmation.

DEVICES AND INNOVATION OF (YOGA VIDHI)

In yoga, mind has numerous levels: mudha (dull and latent psyche), kshipta (occupied brain), vikshipta (mostly diverted psyche), ekagrata (concentrated psyche) and niruddha (controlled psyche).

At the point when we become apparent, our attention is drawn by the view of the psychological examples as the spin (Chitta-vritti) which is five collapsed and comprises of pramana (origination), viparyaya (confusion), vikalpa (creative mind), Nidra (rest) and smrithi (memory)

"Yoga is the stillness of the whirlpools of the mind (yogash chittavritti nirodhah - I: 2). Once this is accomplished, the yogis rest in their essential being (tada drishtu swarupevasthanam - I: 3). The method of achieving this state is through dedicated and purposeful and dispassionate practice (abyasa vairagyabhyam tannirodhah - I: 12, Patanjali - Yoga Darshana).

The yogi sees his being as a manifestation of the divine and realizes that it is not only physical existence, but also has four other levels of reality, including the energy body, the mental body, the body of wisdom, and the body of eternal cosmic bliss. This concept is known as Pancha Kosha.

The yogi follows an orderly practice (Abyasa) of the eightfold method comprising of the ethical limitations (Yama), moral observances (Niyama), firm and agreeable stances (Asana), development of the fundamental life power (Pranayama), control of the faculties (Pratyahara), insightful fixation (Dharana) driving into reflection (Dhyana) and the condition of astronomical cognizance (Samadhi).

Yoga implies restrained and devoted practice (Abyasa), dispassion (Vairagya), and perspicacity (Viveka). Yoga professional endeavors to join together (Yuj) his individual self (Jivatma) with the all-inclusive self (Paramatma).

THE TRUE PURPOSE OF YOGA

The genuine motivation behind this 5,000+-year-old practice was never about bending into the ideal posture, wearing charming yoga outfits, or building Instagram supporters with provocative backbend photographs.

Nowadays, it appears as though everybody is a "yogi." Whether via web-based networking media, enormous pharma-supported TV ads, or innumerable Bikram, hot, and center force studios in each significant city over the globe, yoga has immediately gotten implanted in our standard culture. Thank heavens! It implies we're going the correct way as development, advancing ceaselessly from pure materiality and towards an increasingly careful, empathetic, and otherworldly society. In any case, yoga is about much more than physical ability, mysterious adaptability, or in all honesty – having the ideal yoga goods.

As per Paramahansa Yogananda, writer of top-rated book Autobiography of a Yogi as of late included in the Netflix film Awake and who acquired yoga toward the West 1920 with the Self-Realization Fellowship, "numerous individuals consider yoga simply physical activities — the asanas or stances that have increased broad ubiquity in late decades — yet these are in reality just the most shallow parts of this significant study of unfurling the unending capability of the human psyche and soul." According to Yogananda, humankind had restricted information on the powers that run the universe, so the majority of the higher systems of Yoga were minimal comprehended or polished.

Today, a comprehension of science is quickly changing how we see ourselves and the world. The customary materialistic origination of life as we probably are aware it is rapidly disappearing with the revelation that issue and vitality are one. From Einstein's relativity hypothesis to the ascent of quantum material science, it is the necessary information that each current substance can be decreased to an example or type of vitality, which communicates and interconnects with different structures. A portion of the present most commended physicists even go above and beyond, distinguishing cognizance as the essential ground of all being. In this way, present-day science is currently affirming the good old standards of Yoga rehearsed more than 5,000 years, which certify that solidarity infests the whole Universe.

As indicated by Webster's word reference, the meaning of yoga is:

1. A Hindu mystical way of thinking showing the concealment of all movement of body, mind, and will all together that oneself may understand its differentiation from them and accomplish freedom.

2. An arrangement of activities for achieving substantial or mental control and prosperity." In Sanskrit, The word yoga itself signifies "association": of the individual awareness or soul with the more extensive Universal Consciousness or Spirit.

True Yoga: Beyond the Body

For some professionals, the control of yoga fixates just on Hatha, or physical asana stances. The training starts with twisting or controlling the body, and is centered around the sentiments, or sense-driven wonders the sensory system creates subsequently. At the point when done routinely, the physical act of yoga can help decrease pressure and lift fixation, in general wellbeing, and a feeling of prosperity. Albeit adjusted welfare and well-being are a significant advance towards illumination, it is vital not to mistake this for a definitive motivation behind yoga: setting up the body for contemplation. When the anxiety of the body has been quieted through asana practice, the cognizance would now be able to be coordinated internally to the spirit, which lies past the faculties and material mindfulness. Missing this following stage of training, the experience of yoga can be constrained to the domain of substantial sensations, similar to sex, medications, liquor, or chocolate.

A miserable, however strong case of the restrictions of a body-centered yoga practice is the ongoing sex outrage and court judgment against Bikram Choudhury, the 73-year old author of the more sultry than hot overall Bikram Yoga development. Bikram, or "hot yoga," includes an hour and a half arrangement of 26 yoga presents rehearsed carefully in a muggy 95–108 °F condition. In spite of driving incalculable fans to more quality, adaptability, and prosperity, and making a compelling 75 million dollar realm dependent on physical yoga presents – he still can't seem to pay any of the $6.8 million granted a year ago to his previous lawyer, who charges he explicitly annoyed and afterward terminated her after she examined assault claims from different understudies. Even though he, despite everything, denies the cases, the embarrassment raises doubt about the potential restrictions of a physical-just yoga practice – regardless of how mainstream.

Unaccompanied by more elevated levels of an association through contemplation and control of the body-bound detects, the act of physical yoga resembles taking an hour and a half to set up a tasty, sustaining, full dinner – at that point tossing it in the garbage without tasting it.

Whenever you complete your yoga asana practice, sit still. Ruminate. Turn internal, and permit yourself a minute to taste the profound delight you've endeavored to develop.

THIS IS THE GENUINE MOTIVATION BEHIND YOGA.

Integration of yoga and modern medication

Today we are confronted with various crippling incessant sicknesses identified with maturing, condition, and indulgent way of life, for example, malignant growth, diabetes, osteoporosis, cardiovascular illnesses, AIDS. Current clinical progressions give the justification to the mix of different conventional recuperating strategies, including yoga to advance mending, wellbeing, and life span. The relic of yoga can supplement the cutting edge medication. From the start, allopathic medicines and yoga may appear to be inconsistent. Specialists of either framework are regularly found at loggerheads with each other in the commonplace present-day need to feel superior. It is significantly more straightforward to gather a structure among Yoga and Ayurveda as both offer various resemblances of thoughts, for instance, the Trigunas, Tridoshas, Chakras (imperativeness centers) and Nadis (essentialness channels). They likewise share the understanding that a sound harmony between body, psyche, and soul prompts total wellbeing. Diet and conduct are given significance in the two frameworks, and a definitive objective of both is the fulfillment of Samadhi (solidarity).

There are many gathering focuses on the development of a stable scaffold among yoga and current medication. Both present-day medicine and yoga comprehend the requirement for total wellbeing. Indeed, even the World Health Organization has, as of late, added another measurement to the cutting edge comprehension of wellbeing by remembering profound wellbeing for its meaning of the "condition of wellbeing." Current medication has a definitive point of delivering a condition of ideal physical and psychological wellness in this manner, at last, prompting the perfect prosperity of the person. Yoga likewise focuses on the accomplishment of mental and physical well-being; however, the system differs.

While present-day medication has a great deal to offer mankind in its treatment and the executives of significant ailment, mishaps, and transferable infections, yoga has a ton to provide regarding preventive, promotive and rehabilitative techniques notwithstanding numerous administration strategies to handle current sicknesses while present-day science searches externally for a reason for all ills, the yogi look through the profundity of his self. The potential and show coordination of yoga and present-day clinical science can be examined:

Anatomy and Physiology: The investigation of life structures and physiology is an excellent gathering point for present-day medication and Yoga. Yoga specialists and professionals can profit by the multifaceted and end by point 'separate investigation' of current drug where the body is separated into numerous frameworks, at that point into multiple organs, various tissues lastly into billions of cells. Then again, the all-encompassing yogic perspective on the Pancha Kosha (the five sheathed presence) can enable present-day specialists to understand that we are, 'one-body' living beings yet have four new bodies that are similarly significant. We have the physical body as well as a vitality body, a psychological body, a group of intelligence, and an assortment of endless happiness. A comprehension of the mystic life systems and physiology of Nadis, Chakras, and Bindu's when combined with the useful understanding of the subtleties of the physical body can motivate certain information on the self in all human services workforce.

Avoidance of infection: Modern medication focuses on the significance of restraint; however, the job of preventive medicine is still extremely constrained. The yogic way of life that incorporates the Yama and Niyama can help forestall numerous cutting edge illnesses. Neatness that is educated through Saucha can help prevent and limit the spread of infectious and irresistible sicknesses. Mental harmony and right perspectives of yoga, for example, Pratipaksha Bhavanam (taking the contrary view), Samatvam (the poise of brain) and Vairagya (impartial separation) can help forestall a significant number of the psychosomatic sicknesses going out of control in the cutting edge world. If these yogic qualities just as practices of Asanas, Pranayamas, Kriyas, and Dhyana are instilled in the cutting edge human race, we can forestall numerous ailments that proliferate today.

Advancement of wellbeing: Yoga is a fantastic apparatus for the promotion of welfare. The act of yoga prompts the effective working of the body with homeostasis through the improved functioning of the psycho-immuno-neuro-endocrine framework. A reasonable balance between the thoughtful and parasympathetic wings of the autonomic sensory system prompts an exceptional condition of wellbeing. The World Health Organization (WHO) characterizes wellbeing as a condition of complete physical, mental, and social prosperity and not merely nonattendance of sickness or illness. WHO has additionally, as of late recommended, the fourth element of otherworldly wellbeing; however, it has missed the mark concerning characterizing it without mistaking it for religion.

From a yogic point of view, it's delighting that the WHO definition offers significance to 'prosperity' that is a crucial part of 'being' sound just as 'feeling' solid. There is no utilization in a specialist telling patients that every one of their examinations is 'ordinary' when the patients themselves are not feeling 'great.' This individual part of wellbeing is something that yoga has thought about significant for a considerable number of years. The meaning of asana given in the Yoga Sutra as sthira sukham suggests this condition of consistent prosperity at all degrees of presence (sthira sukham asanam - Yoga Darshan II:46, Patanjali).

Patanjali likewise discloses to us that through the act of asana, we can accomplish an express that is past dualities prompting a quiet and peaceful condition of prosperity (tato dvandva anabhighata - Yoga Darshan II: 48, Patanjali). Yoga targets empowering the person to achieve and keep up a dynamic sukha sthanam that might be characterized as a unique feeling of physical, mental, and profound prosperity.

The World Health Organization (WHO) describes prosperity as a state of complete physical, mental, and social thriving and not only nonattendance of disease or affliction. WHO has likewise lately proposed the fourth element of profound wellbeing yet has missed the mark concerning characterizing it without mistaking it for religion. From a Yogic standpoint, it is gladdening that the WHO definition offers significance to 'prosperity' that is a fundamental part of 'being' sound just as 'feeling' solid. There is no utilization in a specialist telling patients that every one of their examinations is 'typical' when the patients themselves are not feeling 'admirably.' This individual part of wellbeing is something that yoga has thought about significant for a massive number of years. The meaning of asana given in the Yoga Sutra as sthira sukham infers this condition of consistent prosperity at all degrees of presence (sthira sukham asanam - Yoga Darshan II:46, Patanjali).

Patanjali additionally discloses to us that through the act of asana, we can achieve an express that is past dualities prompting a quiet and tranquil condition of prosperity (tato dvandva anabhighata - Yoga Darshan II: 48, Patanjali). Yoga targets empowering the person to accomplish and keep up a dynamic sukha sthanam that might be characterized as a unique feeling of physical, mental, and otherworldly prosperity.

The Bhagavad Gita characterizes yoga as samatvam meaning in this way that yoga is poise at all levels (yogasthah kurukarmani sangam tyaktva dhananjaya siddiyasidhyoh samobutva samatvam yoga uchyate). This might be likewise comprehended as an ideal condition of wellbeing wherein physical homeostasis, and mental serenity happens in a reasonable and sound congruity. One of the primary lacunae of the WHO definition lies in the utilization of the term 'express' that infers wellbeing is something to be accomplished 'for the last time' with no requirement for care about it from that point. If welfare is to be comprehended as a 'state,' at that point, it must be understood as a powerful expression that changes from every day and regularly from minute-to-minute. It is frequently, in reality, all the more testing to keep up this dynamic condition of wellbeing than to try and accomplish it in any case.

The executives of maladies and disarranges: Yoga doesn't discredit the utilization of medications and different strategies for present-day medicines. No yoga advisor should attempt to treat an acute myocardial localized necrosis or an unconscious mishap casualty by yoga systems alone. A harmonious connection between the strategies of present-day medication and yoga can help the patient over a one-sided refusal to see the 'opposite side.'

Yoga has a great deal to offer regarding psychosomatic scatters and in stress-related disarranges, for example, diabetes, asthma, bad-tempered inside disorder, epilepsy, hypertension, back agony, and other pragmatic issues. Yoga can help diminish and now and again wipe out medication measurements and reliance on patients experiencing diabetes mellitus, hypertension, epilepsy, nervousness, bronchial asthma, obstruction, dyspepsia, a sleeping disorder, joint inflammation, sinusitis, and dermatological issue. Asanas are likely the best instrument to upset any educated examples of wrong substantial endeavors. Pranayama and Pratyahara are amazingly effective strategies to redirect the person's consideration from the objects of the external condition, to build each individual's vitality possibilities, and to 'interiorize' them, to accomplish control of one's inward working.

Yoga specialists must work a couple with clinical specialists when they are treating patients who have been on allopathic treatment. There are numerous examples where the patient stops clinical treatment imagining that it is not any more essential as they have begun yoga. Undesirable responses could be handily kept away from by pair discussions of yoga advisor and clinical master. Numerous cutting edge specialists will, in general, prescribe the patient to take up yoga and unwinding systems and neglect to refer to the yoga advisor what they really need the patients to do. Most allopathic meds should be decreased dynamically as opposed to being halted out of nowhere. We frequently discover this slip-up as to corticosteroids just as heart prescriptions where unexpected stoppage can be destructive. We should recollect Plato's words when he stated, "The treatment of the part shouldn't be endeavored without a treatment of the sum," implying that the treatment of the body without treating the psyche and soul would be futile.

Rehabilitation: Yoga as a type of exercise based recuperation has a great deal to offer patients of physical and mental impairments. A significant number of the acts of physiotherapy and other exercise-based recuperations share a great deal practically speaking with yoga rehearses. The mix of yoga and non-intrusive treatments can profit patients with learning incapacities. Musculoskeletal issues can be treated by the combination to improve work just as scope of development, quality, and continuance capacities. The blend treatment can likewise improve equalization and finesse. Yoga practice can help those recuperating from mishaps and physical injuries to financially recover quicker and with better useful capacity. Yoga additionally has a great deal to offer those experiencing medication and substance maltreatment in helping them to return to typical life. Yoga builds up their poise and self-control, and furthermore gives them another way of thinking of living; This is fundamental as else they will slip by into their old negative propensities.

Healthy eating regimen: This is a spot that advanced medication and yoga can help give a patient just as should be expected individual the best possible all-encompassing estimations of an appropriate eating routine. Present-day inquire about shows us the advantages of the 'separate' investigation of nourishments based on their physical and synthetic properties. This is significant for the individual to know the amount of every constituent of nourishment is to be taken in the correct amount. Yoga can assist an individual with learning the proper demeanor towards food just as comprehend ideas dependent on the Trigunas and Tridoshas for better wellbeing. Yoga instructs us that the reason for most malady is through under (Ajjeranatvam), over (Atijeeranatvam), or wrong (Kujeeranatvam) absorption. Yoga additionally shows us the way to deal with nourishment, the kinds of food just as the significance of timings, and control in the diet. A blend of the cutting edge parts of the diet with a portion of the yogic idea can support the correct eating routine. Yoga underscores the significance of eating the exact kind of nourishment as well as the perfect sum and with the correct mentality. Importance of not eating alone, just as readiness and serving of food with adoration, are brought out in the yogic plan of the right living. Guna (innate nature) of nourishment is thought about to achieve and keep up great wellbeing. The present-day study of diet can gain so much from this old idea of the arrangement of food as indicated by inherent nature as it is a wholly dismissed part of the current eating regimen.

"He who eats after the past feast has been processed needs no medication." (marunthuena vaendaavaam yaakkaikku arundiyathu atrathu poatri unnin - Tirukkural 942). He likewise says that life in the body turns into a delight if we eat nourishment to stomach related measure (attraal alavuarinthu Unga aghduudambu pettraan nedithu uikkum aaru - Tirukkural 943).

Unwinding: Modern medication comprehends the significance of unwinding for stable living. The issue is that, however, the specialist advises the patient to relax, they don't disclose to them how to do as such, and possibly in truth, they don't have the foggiest idea about the appropriate response themselves. Hatha Yoga and Jnana Yoga unwinding rehearse help loosen up the body and brain. Unwinding is a critical component of any yoga treatment routine and must not be overlooked at any expense. Shavasana has been accounted for to support a great deal in hypertensive patients and practices, for example, Savitri Pranayama, Chandra Pranayama, Kaya Kriya, Yoga Nidra, Anuloma Viloma Prakriyas and Marmanasthanam Kriya are likewise accessible to the individual requiring this condition of complete unwinding. Remember that unwinding all alone is less compelling than unwinding that follows Asanas (stances), for example, dynamic physical effort.

Adapting aptitudes: Yoga has a great deal to offer the individuals who can't adapt to death and biting the dust just as those experiencing hopeless sicknesses. The yoga theory of living considers demise to be an unavoidable part of life that can't be wished away. The individuals who are dealing with the perishing just as those dealing with patients of severe sicknesses and significant handicaps are under an extraordinary measure of pressure and yoga practice only as its way of thinking encourages them to gain the inward quality essential to carry out their responsibility. Yoga can help break the horrendous winding of agony medicate measurement torment and, by doing so, help decrease the medication dose in patients enduring incessant pain. It has been accounted for that yoga improves personal satisfaction in patients experiencing malignant growth and causes them to adapt better with the impacts of treatment. It loosens up them and encourages them to rest better.

Consumption: Modern medication is frequently censured for the cost engaged with its techniques for treatment. Yoga offers an economic strategy for wellbeing that can be added to the clinical ordnance when required. Yoga just requires the patient's exertion (will) and genuinely needn't bother with any gear. The cutting edge yoga industry would prefer to have us accept that we need huge amounts of yoga gear to begin yoga. Decrease in tranquilize measurements and shirking of pointless medical procedures, as a rule, can likewise help lessen the spiraling expense of medicare.

The procedure of maturing: Aging is inescapable, and yoga can assist us with aging smoothly. Current medication attempts to help hinder maturing and assist individuals with looking better by exorbitant careful strategies that are just an outside covering over the fundamental maturing process. Healthy eating regimen, normal exercise, shirking of negative propensities, and development of the positive tendencies and a reliable way of life can assist us with aging with pride. Yoga can likewise help our 'silver residents' hold their psychological capacity and forestall degenerative clutters. Physical mishaps, for example, falls can be limited, and numerous an artificial hip, knee, or shoulder substitution medical procedure can be kept away from.

Psychotherapy: In the field of psychotherapy and therapy, we can discover a ton of antiquated yogic ideas being repeated on numerous occasions. Numerous advanced psychotherapeutic approaches, for example, ID, projection, and transference, are like ideas in yoga brain science. Yoga brain research incorporates differing standards inside a solitary body. "Chakras speak to a genuine exertion to give an emblematic hypothesis of the mind" (Jung, 1999). His 'focal point of character' idea dependent on dream examination is fundamentally the same as the yogic idea of a focal clairvoyant or profound nature. He additionally related chakras to the originals that possess large amounts of the aggregate oblivious Yoga helps the psychotherapist in preparing mindfulness, and in the self guideline of body, diet, breath, feelings, propensity designs, values, will, oblivious weights and drives. It likewise helps in understanding the prototype forms and to a transient being. Yoga offers an incorporated technique as opposed to one that is found in separation in a wide range of treatments. The hypothesis of Kleshas is a magnificent model for psychotherapy, while enthusiastic treatments of yoga incorporate Swadhyaya, Pranayama, Pratyahara, Dharana, Dhyana, and Bhajans. Improvement of legallegal mental perspectives is taught by means of the ideas of Vairagya, Chitta Prasadanam, just as Patanjali's educate on embracing the mentalities regarding Maitri, Karuna, Mudita, and Upekshanam towards the glad, the affliction, the great and the fiendishness disapproved of people. Both yoga and therapy share a shared view in understanding that indications of the illness frequently result in the consideration patters of the patients. While all psychoanalysts must experience analysis themselves, it is instructed in yoga that one should initially experience a profound Sadhana, before endeavoring to manage others on the way. In contrast, analysis looks through the oblivious, yoga endeavors to comprehend and investigate the overly cognizant.

Way of life changes: Yoga places extraordinary significance on an appropriate and solid way of life whose fundamental parts are Achar (sound exercises all the time), Vichar (right contemplations and disposition towards life), Ahar (sound, supporting eating regimen) and Vihar (legitimate recreationaactivitieses to loosen up body and psyche). They figure out how to put forth an attempt and improve their way of life with the goal that their wellbeing can improve. Way of life change is the trendy expression in present-day clinical circles, and yoga can assume an essential job right now. Yogic eating regimen, Asanas, Pranayamas, Mudras, Kriyas, and unwinding are a significant part of the way of life alteration. To carry on with a solid life, it is critical to do sound things and follow a sound way of life.

Women's health: Healthy moms bring forth solid infants, and a sound beginning has an extraordinary future ahead. Yoga, in blend with present-day medication, has a great deal to add to the wellbeing status of womankind. Adolescence and menopause become simpler advances with the assistance of yoga. Pubertal changes have been moderately smoother in yoga specialists than their partners who don't rehearse yoga. The Oli Mudras as rehearsed in the yoga custom have extraordinary potential right now; additionally, the Swara Yoga has a ton of energizing prospects. When origination happens, yoga encourages the youthful mother to set herself up genuinely and intellectually for the up and coming labor. Yoga helps open the joints of the pelvis and hip just as fortify the stomach muscles for labor. Afterward, straightforward Pranayamas and unwinding procedures help the new mother unwind and appreciate the new experience of her life. Baby blues presentation of straightforward practices alongside breathing, unwinding, and a ton of creeping encourages her return to ordinary prior, and this can be utilized in all maternity clinics alongside allopathic administration. Yoga practices can likewise help diminish the medication measurements in clinical issues that regularly confuse a typical pregnancy.

Research: Scientific looks into the field of yoga have an essential essentialness for check of the significance of yoga and improvement of medication, however different sciences, too. Yoga gives outlines for the new understanding and new way to deal with the view of the human wellbeing. Numerous inquires about of the yoga practice benefits are not satisfactorily methodologically developed, and yoga practice of the patients doesn't have support in yoga gauges. The higher parts of yoga are as yet not in the researchable domain of current science; however, it doesn't imply that it won't be. Along these lines, it is essential to examine new methodological instruments for estimating various marvels that impact human presence and advancement.

PRE-YOGA ORIENTATION AND PREPARATION

Before You Start

Before setting out on the yoga plan, you can consult your health or wellness specialist on the off chance that you have an ailment. It also refers to under 12-year-old pregnant women and young people.

The data given inside this book is accepted to be precise, yet the peruser is liable for talking with their wellbeing proficient before changing the eating routine or beginning an activity program; it's anything but a substitute for appropriate clinical guidance. If anything else fails, the primary care physician or certified health professional will be counseling you.

When To Practice

Set aside a specific time in your day to make the most of your Yoga practice. First light and nightfall are viewed as the best times to rehearse Yoga, as the rising and setting of the sun accuse our assortment of exceptional vitality. In any case, if these occasions are unimaginable for you, find some other time that works best for you and practice reliably. Practice in the first part of the day in the event that you need to set up your brain and body for the afternoon, and accuse your assortment of positive vitality. Remember that toward the beginning of the day or in a chilly climate, your muscles will be stiffer, so slip cautiously into the stances at first. Practice at night if you need to unwind following a distressing day, loosen up and focus. In the nighttime, your body will be progressively flexible, so you'll have the option to go further into stances.

Where To Practice

Discover a spot where you are most drastically averse to be upset. It tends to be your room, nursery, or seashore - inside or outside, any place there is an even, flat surface.

On the off chance that you are rehearsing inside, ensure that the room is ventilated and with agreeable temperature. Cooled rooms are not prudent - when the earth is cold, your body is firm, and muscles stretch gradually. A spotless situation and outside air adds extra benefits to the breathing practice.

Ensure that you have enough space to permit you to move around and expand the arms and legs uninhibitedly. Turn your telephone off and balance a note on your entryway to state that you have the opportunity to yourself.

This is YOUR time.

Eating and Drinking

Never practice straightforwardly in the wake of eating. Yoga ought to be done on a void stomach. Accordingly, permit in any event 1 hour after a bite and 2 - 3 hours after an overwhelming supper before you start your training.

It is ideal to drink previously or after your Yoga meeting, to abstain from getting got dried out. Attempt to abstain from drinking water during the training to abstain from losing your focus on Yoga stances and relaxing.

In any case, have a glass of warm water before your workout, or a small bite (organic food or yogurt), on the off chance that you will be rehearsing at the beginning of the day. Have a legal breakfast at the point where you finish your preparation.

What to Wear

Wear agreeable, light, free apparel, ideally made of common fibers. Your garments ought not to limit your developments.

Evacuate your adornments, watch, and display if conceivable. Yoga is practiced with uncovered feet.

What You Need

Get an exceptional Yoga tangle for yourself. It gives cushioning just as a non-slip surface to rehearse on and makes your training simpler and more secure. You can find one in any games shop. Nobody else should utilize your tangle. This isn't just for cleanliness reasons, yet in addition, since you will, in the long run, develop vitality on your tangle that will bolster you all through the Yoga practice.

You can likewise get a pad to make your contemplation increasingly agreeable and a cover if you wish to cover yourself while unwinding in the Corpse Pose toward the finish of the meeting.

On the off chance that you need, you can play unwinding, calming music out of sight - simply ensure it's not very uproarious.

THE MOST EFFECTIVE METHOD TO PRACTICE

Play out all the stances gradually and with control. You are not in rivalry with anybody, not by any means yourself. You'll advance quicker when you take things gradually.

❖ Concentrate on your breathing, feel the air gradually flowing through your body, unwinding and empowering it.

❖ Relax. Relinquish any extra pressure, stress, or negative considerations.

❖ Start each meeting with the warm-up. It's fundamental to dodge wounds.

❖ Modify the stances for your body. The guidelines and photos of the yoga in this book are the final objective - the bearing you are going towards, not where you should be after your first scarcely any meetings. Analysis and investigation of various positions and arrangements to make the stance work for your body.

❖Try not to anticipate immediate results. Yoga is not a fast fix for your weight issues. Persistence is a vital aspect of opening the long haul thinning benefits of Yoga.

❖ Have Fun! An ideal approach to get results with your Yoga practice is to appreciate it. Feeling cheerful while rehearsing Yoga places the psyche and body into a positive state.

❖ Most Importantly, tune in to and regard your body. Never suppress any development. It's your most influential coach; let your body lead you!

Warm-Up Poses

Before the main yoga training commences, a few poses are indulged in to put people in the yoga mood.

Body turn

Instructions

❖ stand straight with your legs separated

❖ breathe in lift the hands from the sides on the shoulder level

❖ breathe out and go to one side in the midsection keeping both the arms and shoulders straight

❖ turn beyond what many would consider possible

❖ breathe in and contort back to the front

- breathe out and contort to the correct side

- this is one round

- rehash once again

Forward/Backward bend

Instructions:

- stand straight with your legs separated

- breathe in welcome your hands on the midsection

- breathe out and twist forward from the midriff keeping the knees straight

- twist down however much as could reasonably be expected

- breathe in and return to starting position

- breathe out and twist in reverse

- breathe in return to starting position

- this is one round

- rehash once again

Side twists

Guidelines:

- stand straight with your legs separated

- breathe in and welcome your hands on the midsection

- breathe out and twist the body in the abdomen to one side

- keep the knees straight

- breathe in and return to the beginning position

- breathe out and twist the body in the abdomen to the correct side

- breathe in and return to starting posture

- this is one round

- rehash once again

Chest area revolutions

Directions:

- stand straight with your legs separated

- breathe in unite your hands over the head

- breathe out and twist forward from the midriff keeping the knees straight

- breathe in pivot your chest area to one side

- keep breathing in and curve to the back

- breathe out and curve to one side

- ❖ keep breathing out and twist forward

- ❖ breathe in and return, pivot to one side

- ❖ continue breathing in and pivot to the back

- ❖ breathe out and turn to one side

- ❖ continue breathing out and turn to the front

- ❖ return to beginning standing posture

- ❖ this is one round

- ❖ rehash once again

Shoulder revolutions

Guidelines:

- ❖ stand straight with your legs separated

- ❖ your hands on the shoulders

- ❖ inhale regularly

- ❖ begin turning your arms in huge circles to the back - 5 circles

- ❖ rehash revolution to the front - 5 circles

- ❖ discharge the hands and return to starting standing posture

Twist rotations

Directions:

❖ stand straight with your legs separated

❖ get your hands front on the shoulder level

❖ Start turning your two wrists.

❖ turn five circles to the external side, at that point 5 circles the other way

❖ discharge the hands and return to beginning standing posture

Head pivots

Directions:

❖ stand straight with your legs separated

❖ welcome your hands on the midriff

❖ twist the neck forward and begin turning to one side, to the back, to one side and front

❖ pivot back to one side, back, left and front

❖ rehash once again

❖ fix the neck and discharge the hands, return to the underlying standing posture

Swinging while at the same time standing posture

Guidelines:

❖ stand straight with your legs separated

❖ Raise your arms above your head, holding the elbows straight

❖ twist forward and swing the storage compartment down from the hips

❖ permit the arms and head to swing through the legs

❖ be sans pressure like a cloth doll

❖ return easily to the upstanding situation with the arms raised

❖ breathe in strongly through the nose while raising the arms and breathe out powerfully while swinging downwards

❖ rehash multiple times

BASIC YOGA POSES

Yoga poses (additionally called Asanas) are physical stances that activity your whole body, stretch and tone the muscles and joints, the spine, and whole skeletal framework. They have a useful impact on the body outline, yet additionally on the inward organs, glands, and nerves, keeping all frameworks sound. Asanas decrease pressure, improve unwinding, and renew body, brain, and spirit.

In this book, you'll be directed through the most significant stances from customary Hatha Yoga that guide in upgrading weight reduction. To make your considering simpler, all stances are composed in indistinguishable gatherings: Standing Poses, Sun Salutation, Balancing Poses, Sitting Poses, etc. Bear as a top priority that I have deliberately kept the directions exceptionally short, to assist you with concentrating on your body and not on my talking. Keep in mind; Yoga is about advancement, not flawlessness. Continue rehearsing, and you will gradually consummate your stances, and this book will be your closest companion en route.

Sun Salutations

Prayer pose

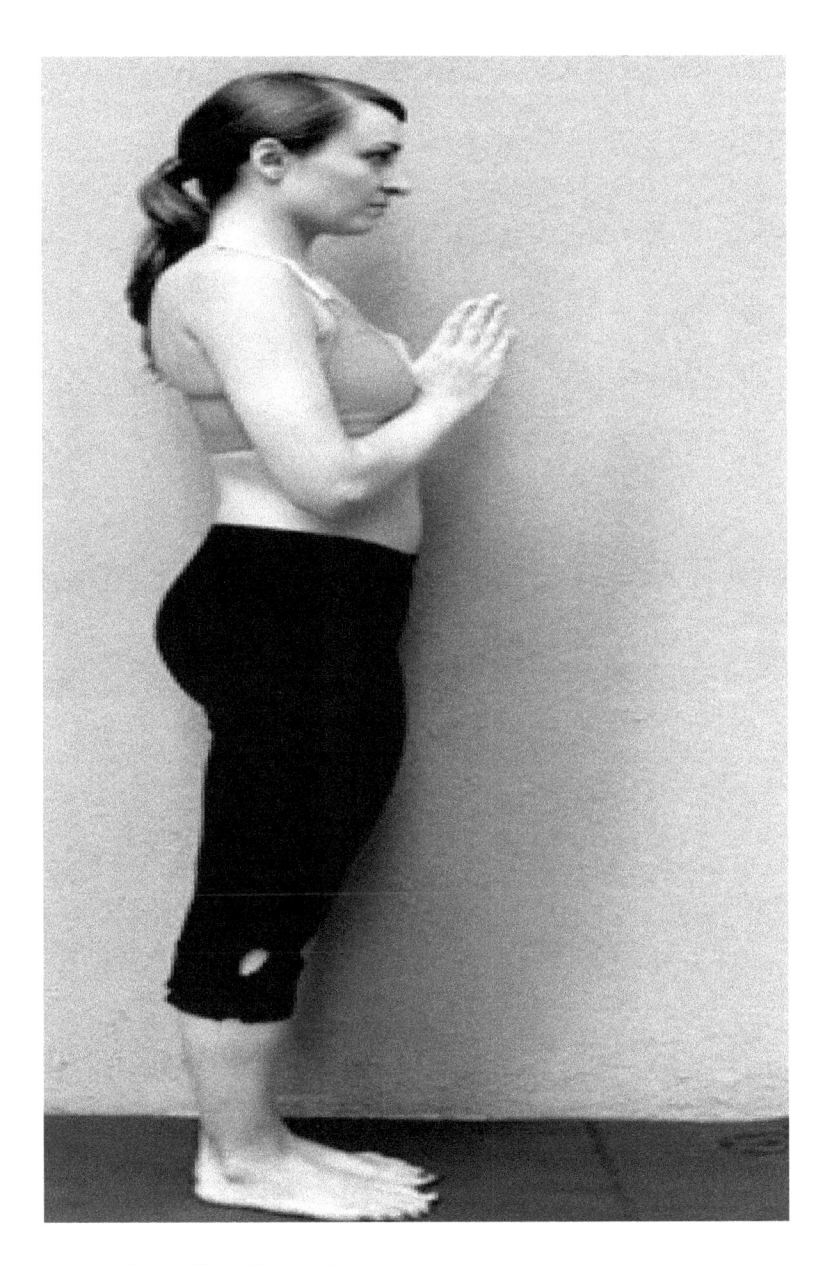

Standing back arch

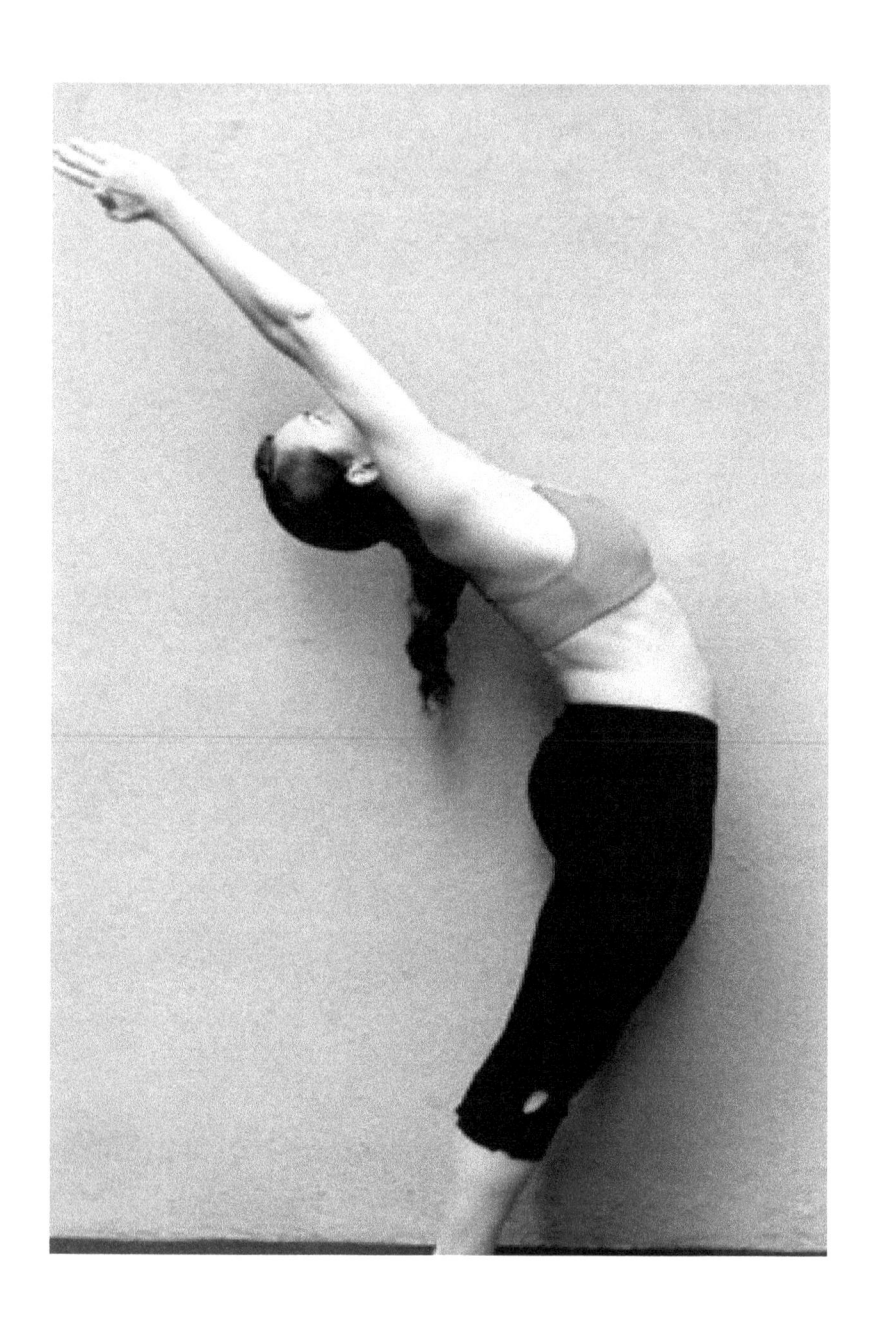

Forward bend

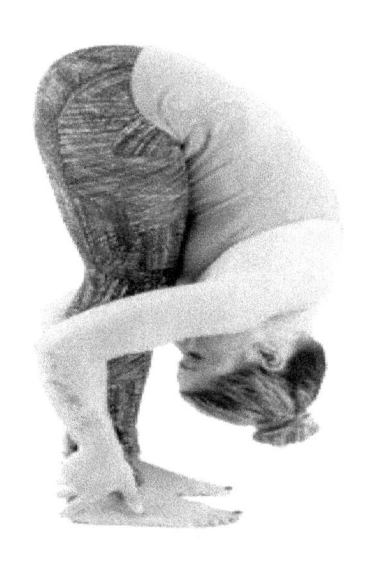

Half cobra pose

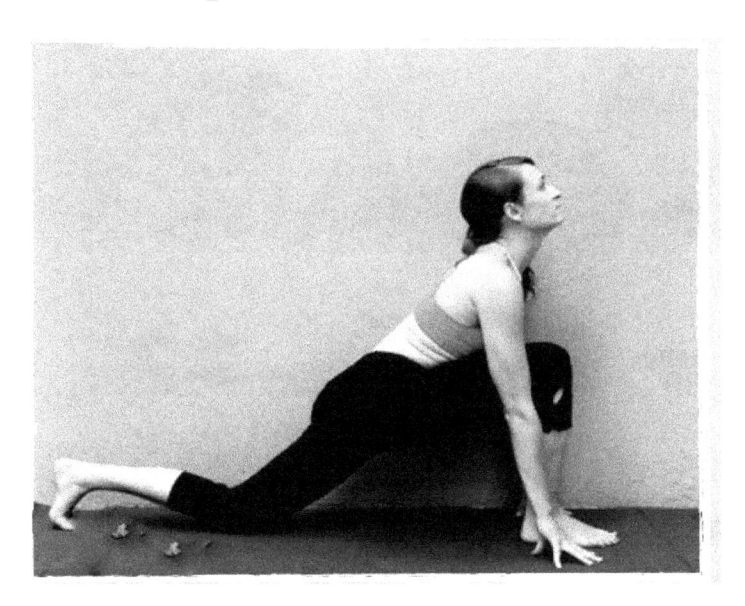

Plank pose

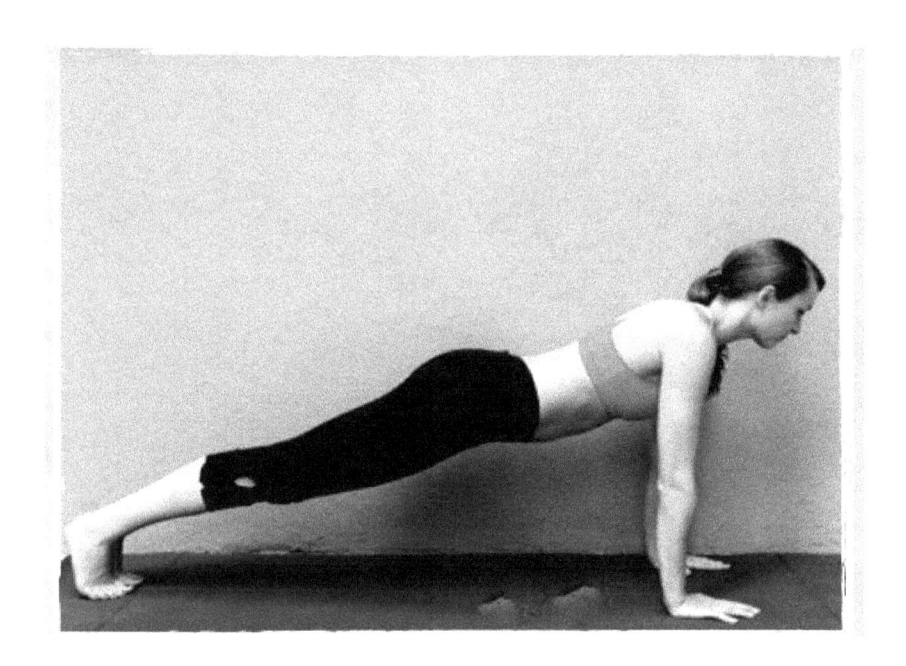

Ashtanga pose

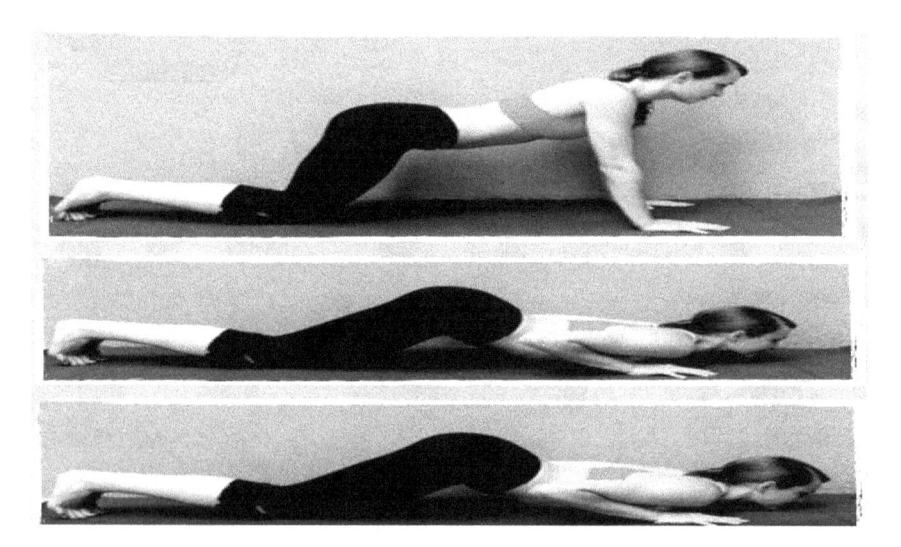

Cobra pose

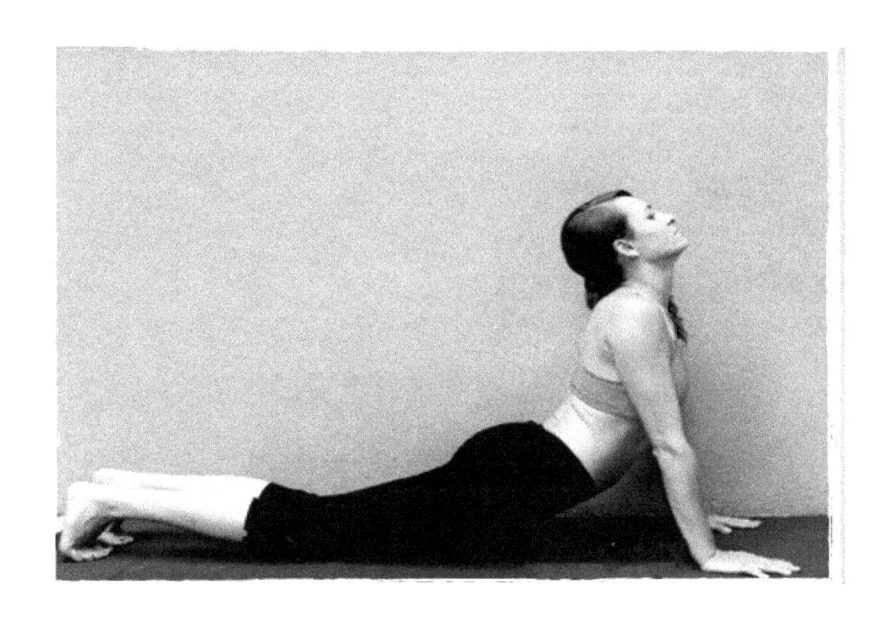

Downward facing dog pose

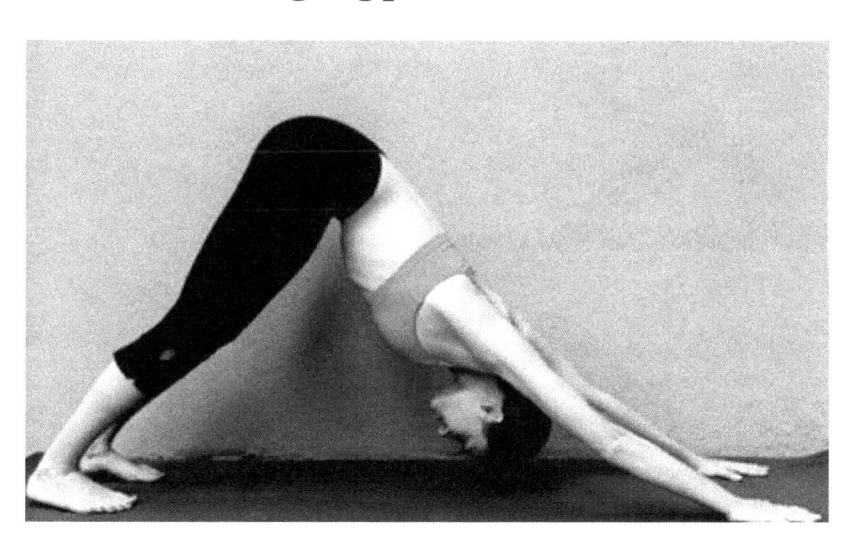

Standing Poses

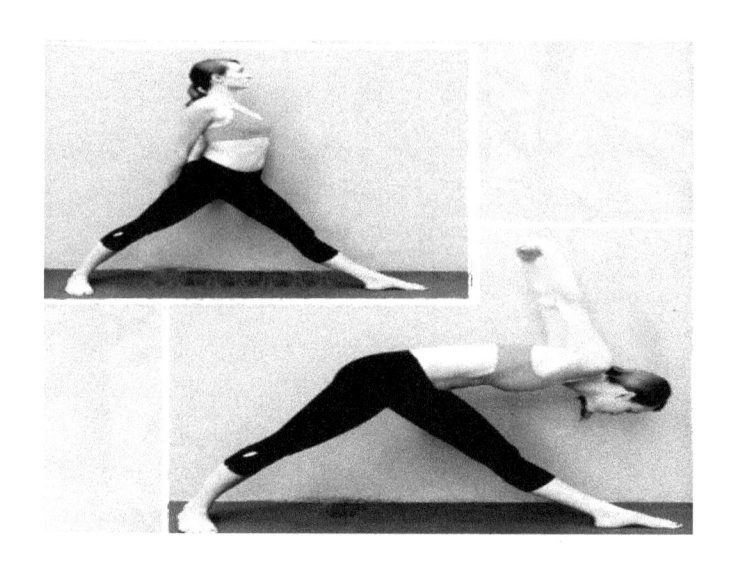

One leg forward bend and Triangle pose

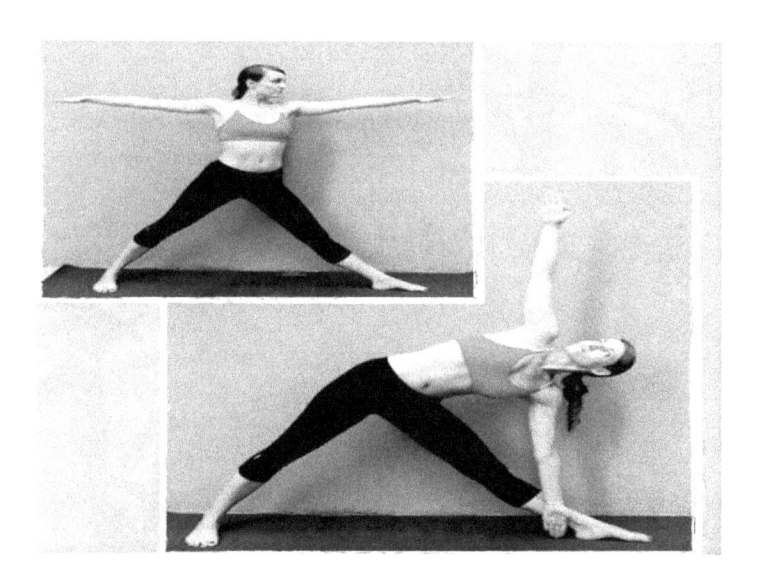

One hand backbend

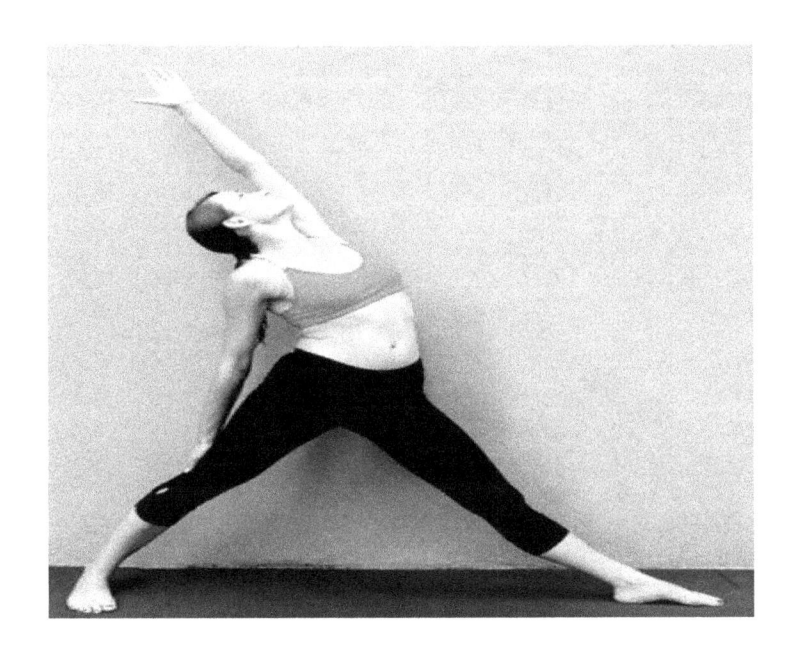

Revolved triangle pose

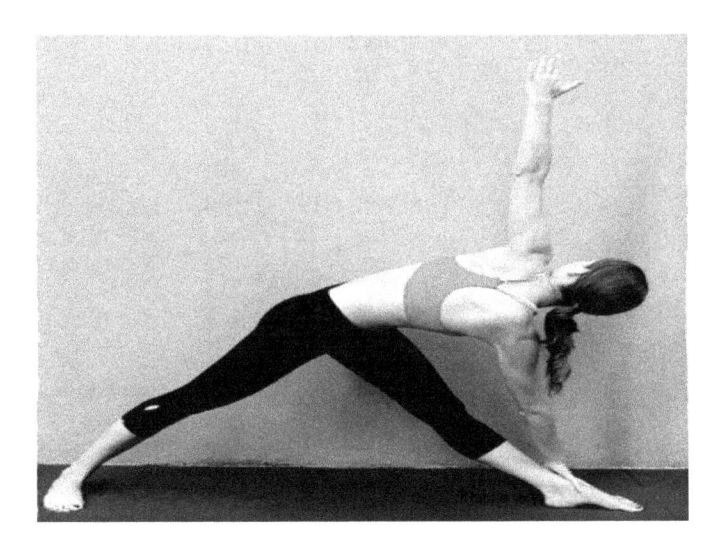

Side angle stretch

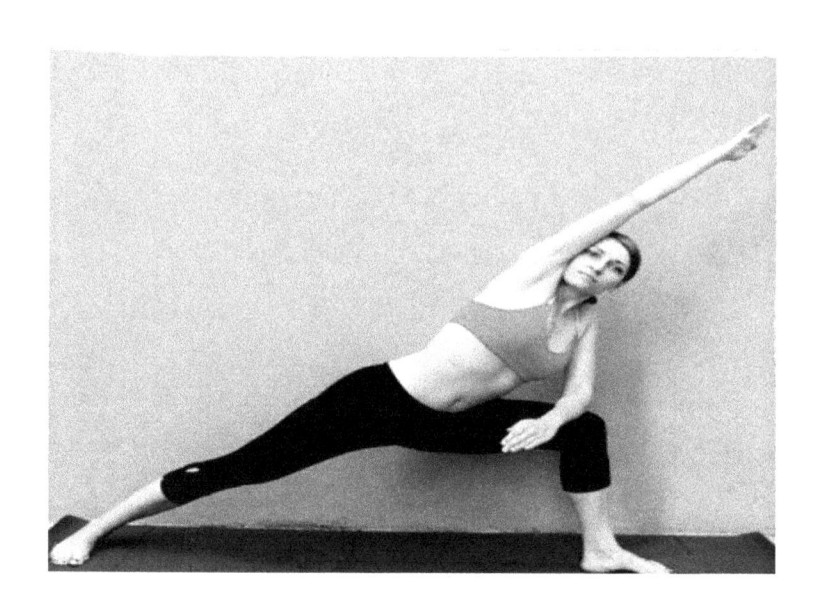

Revolved side angle stretch

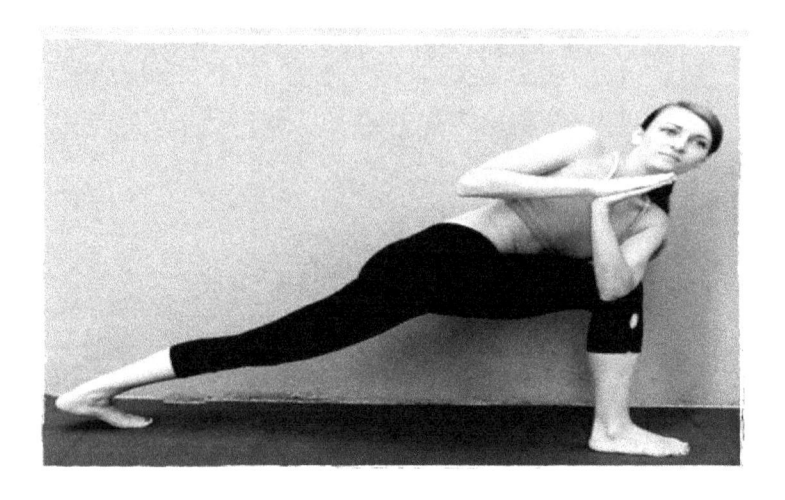

Chest expand

Wide Leg Forward Bend I

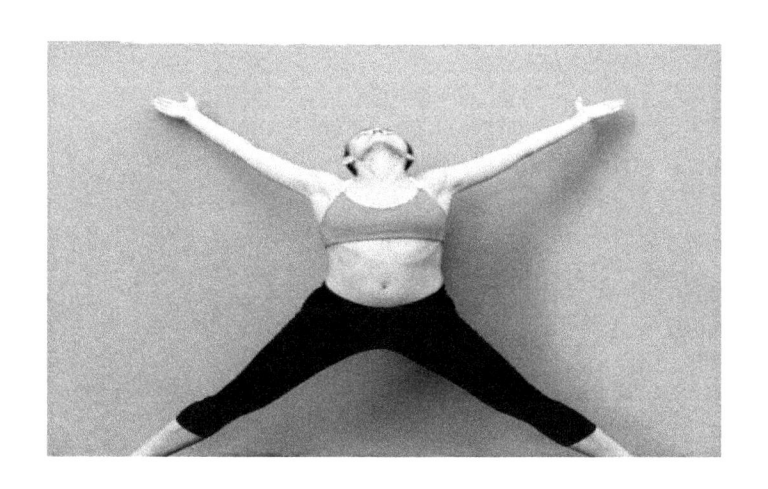

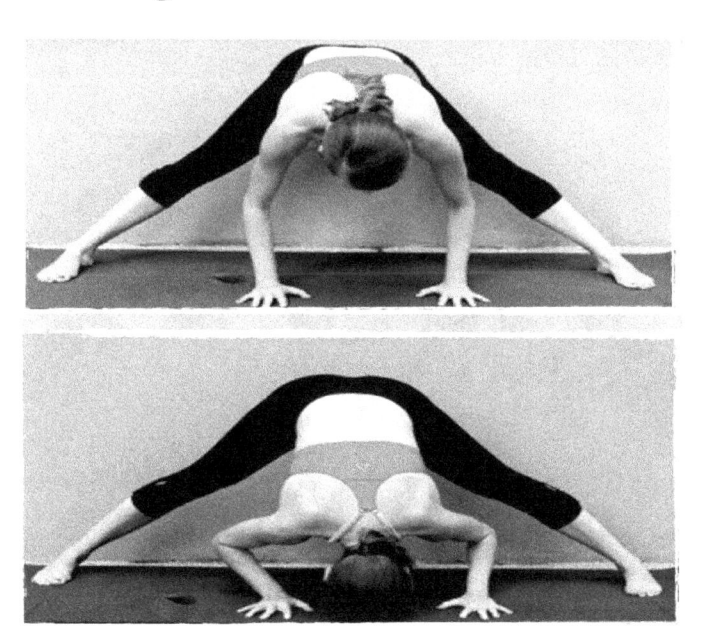

Wide Leg Forward Bend II

Wide Leg Forward Twist

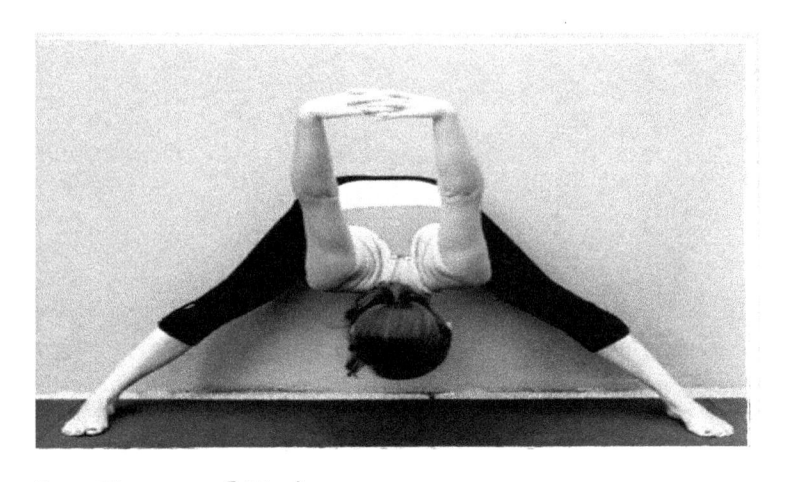

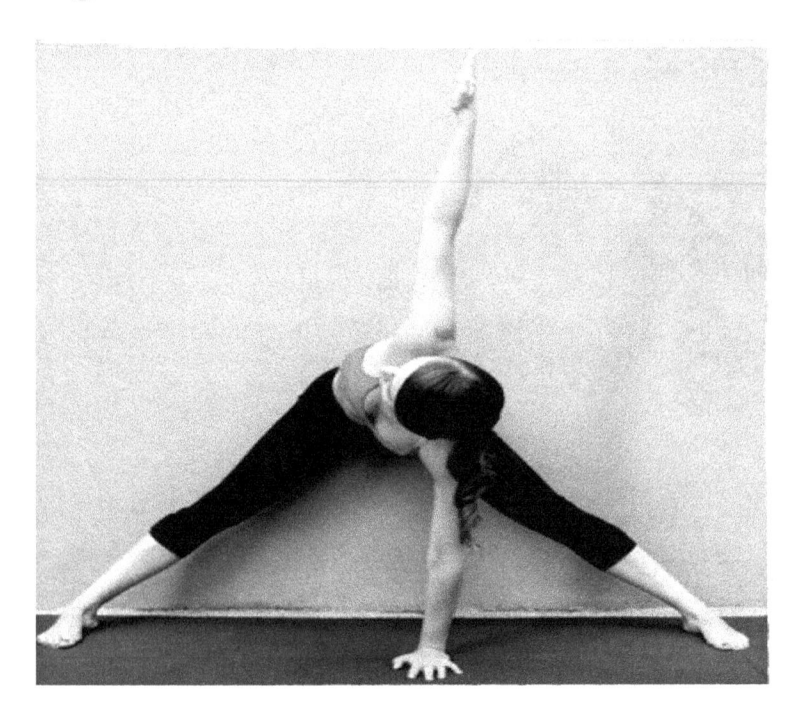

Warrior Pose I

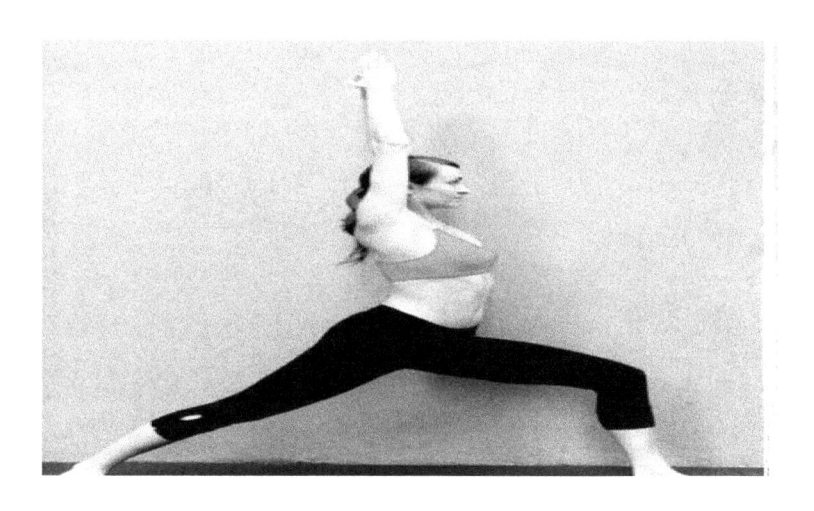

Warrior Pose I and Warrior pose II

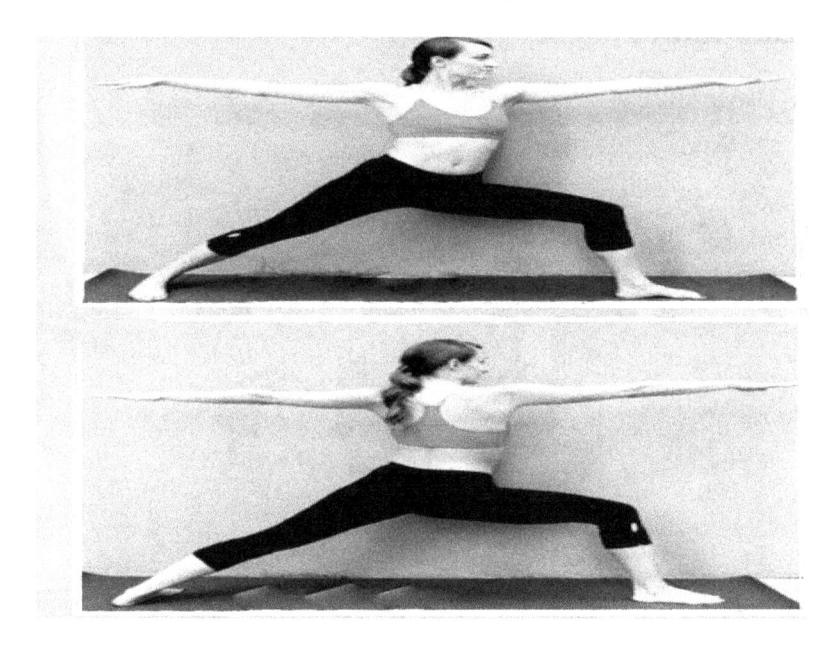

Easy Warrior Pose III

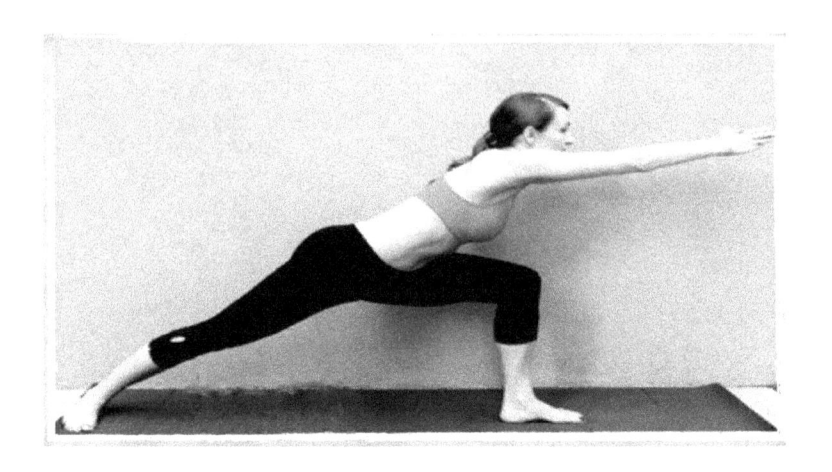

Easy Half Moon Pose

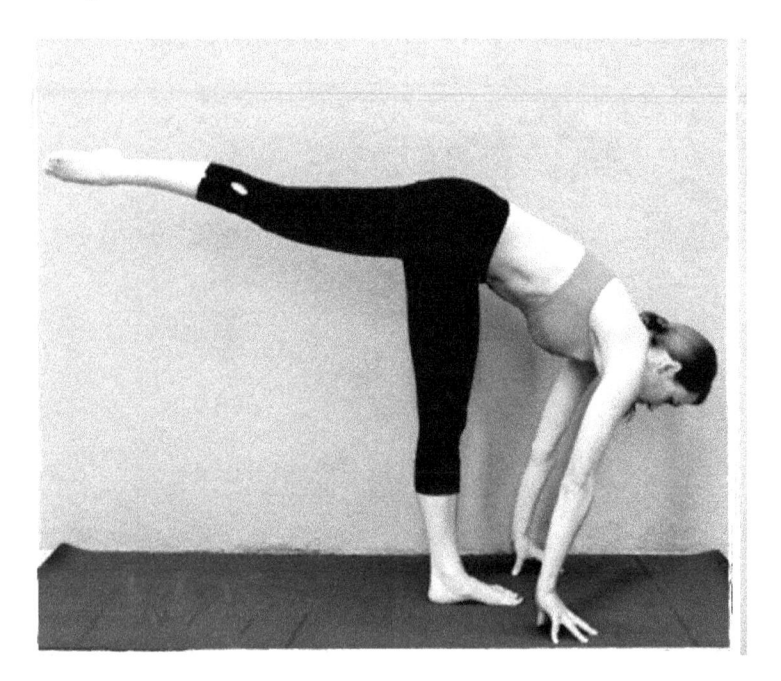

Tree Pose

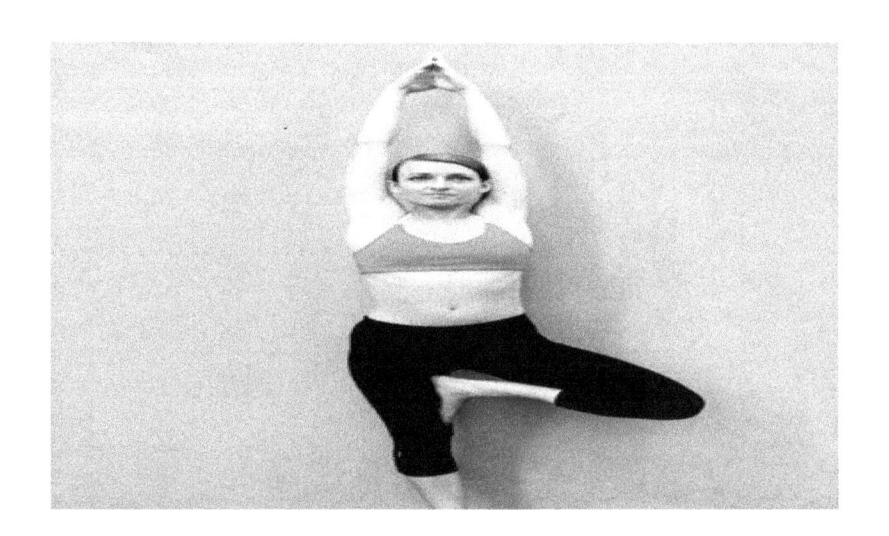

Standing Half Bow Balance

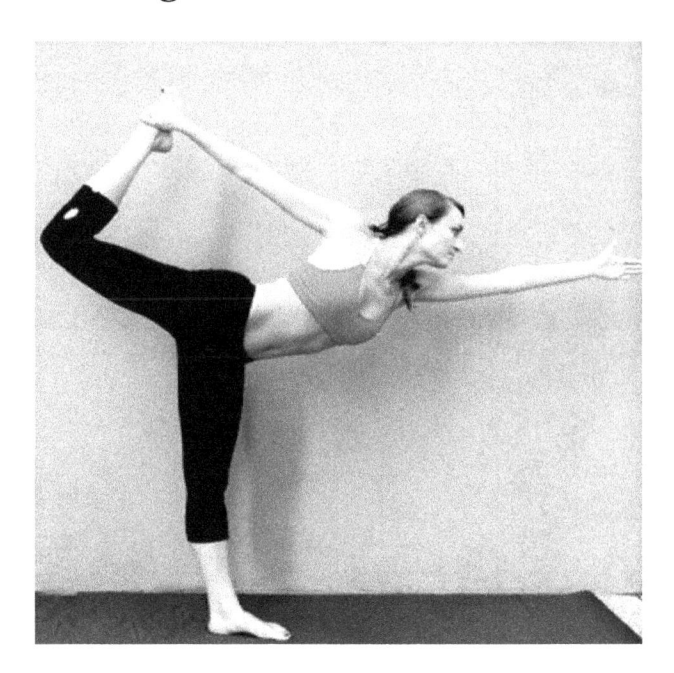

Standing Knee To Chest Balance

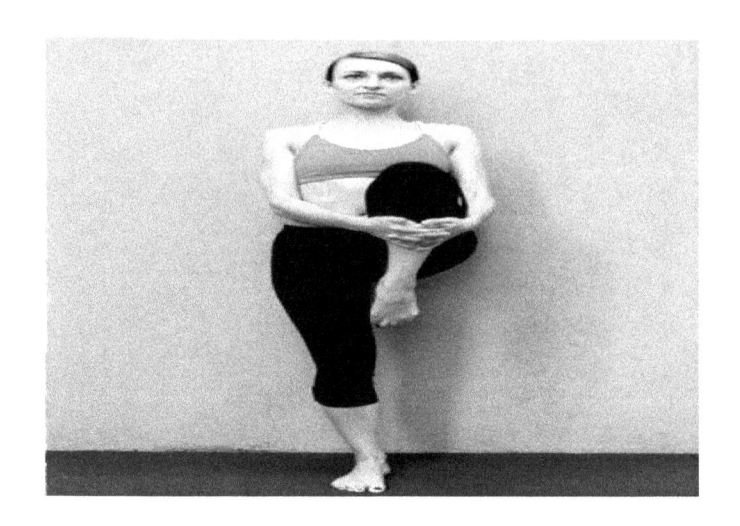

Standing Knee Side Balance

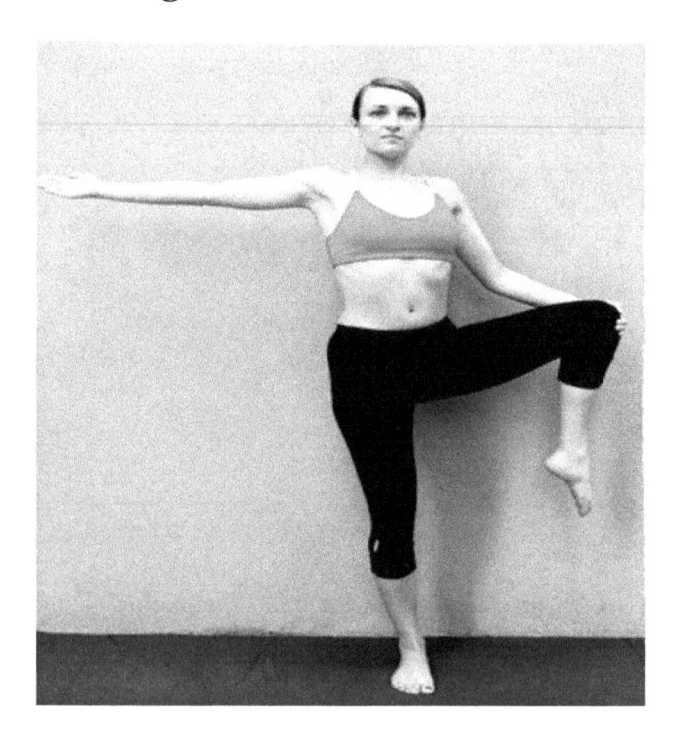

Eagle Pose

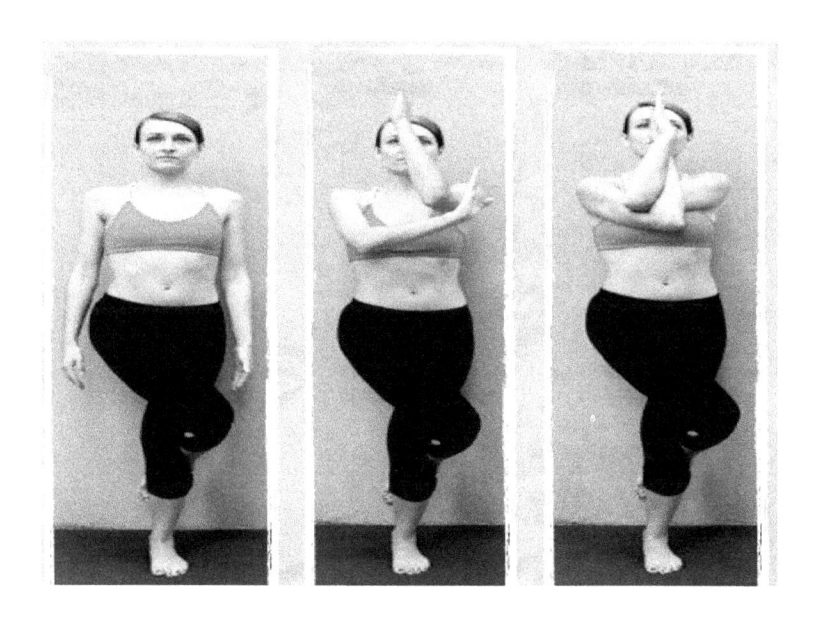

Chair Pose

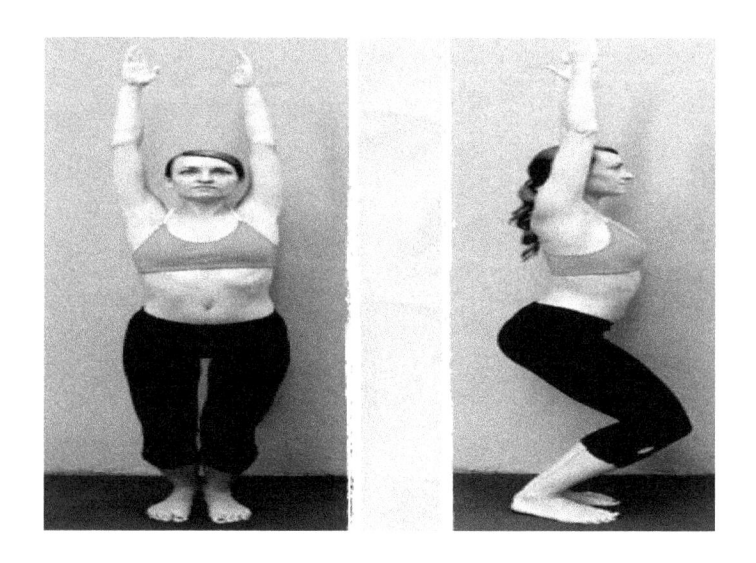

Sitting Poses

Easy Meditation Pose

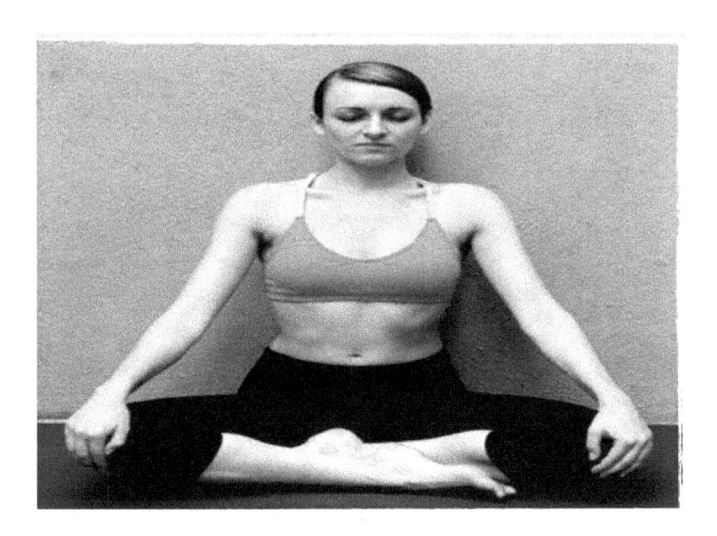

Half Lotus Pose

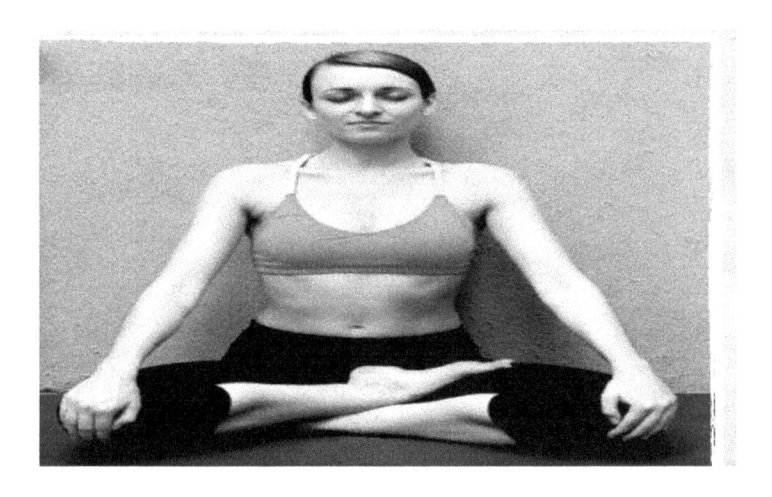

Lotus Pose.

Thunderbolt Pose I

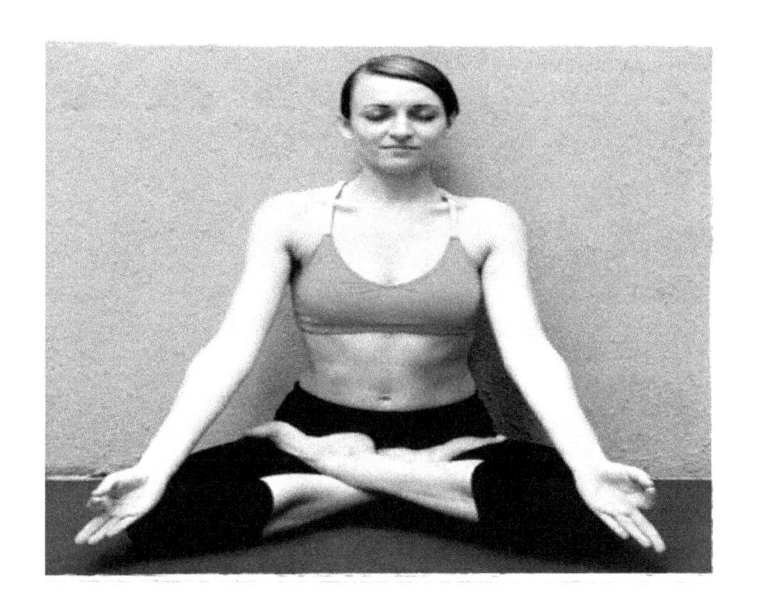

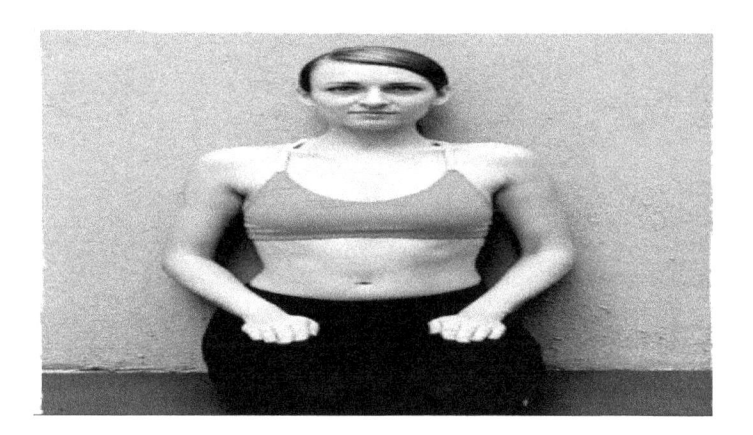

Thunderbolt Pose II

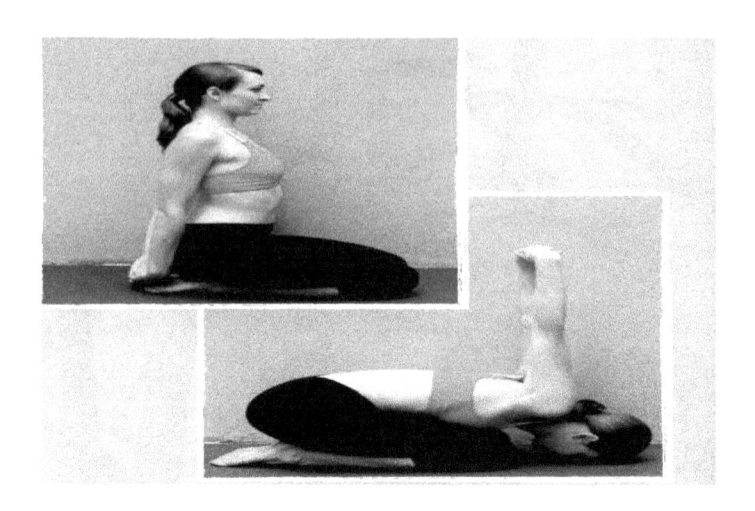

Thunderbolt Pose III

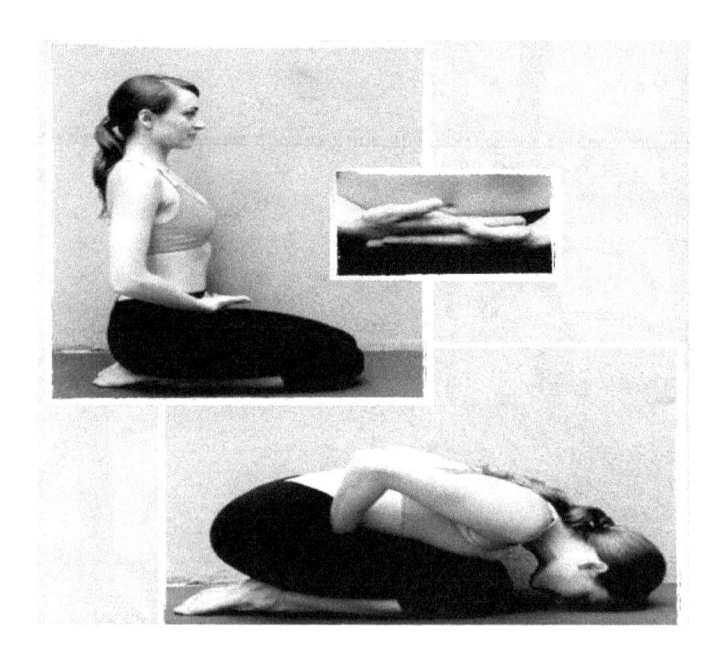

One Leg Forward Bend I

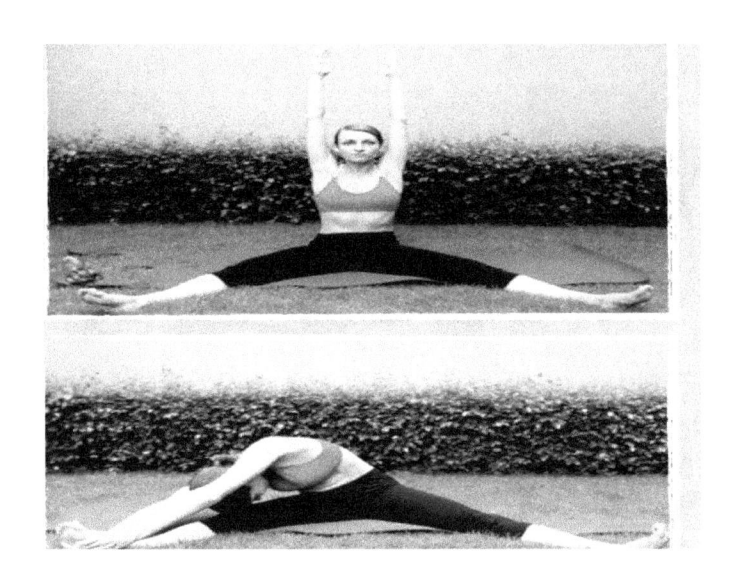

One Leg Forward Bend II

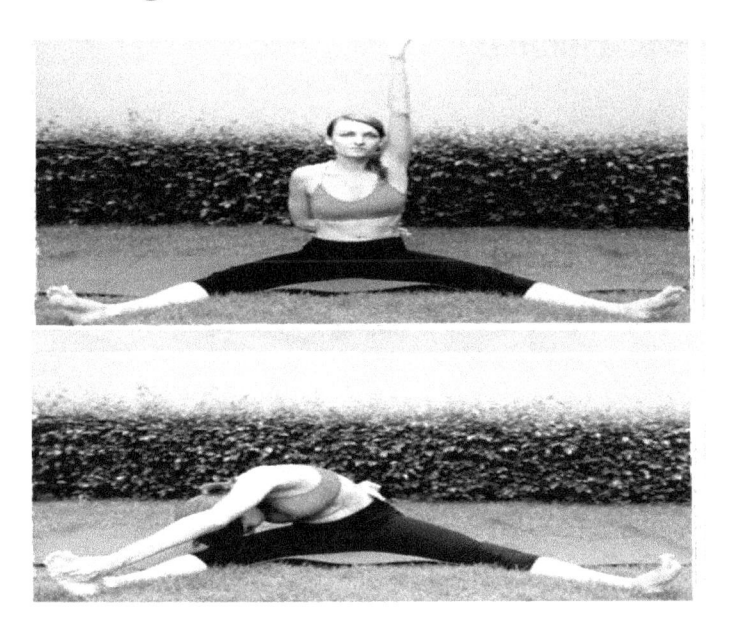

Two Legs Forward Bend I

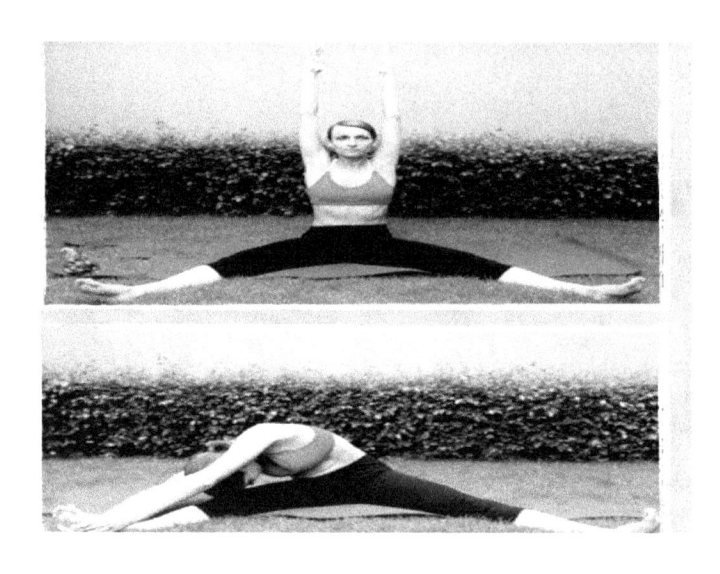

Two Legs Forward Bend II

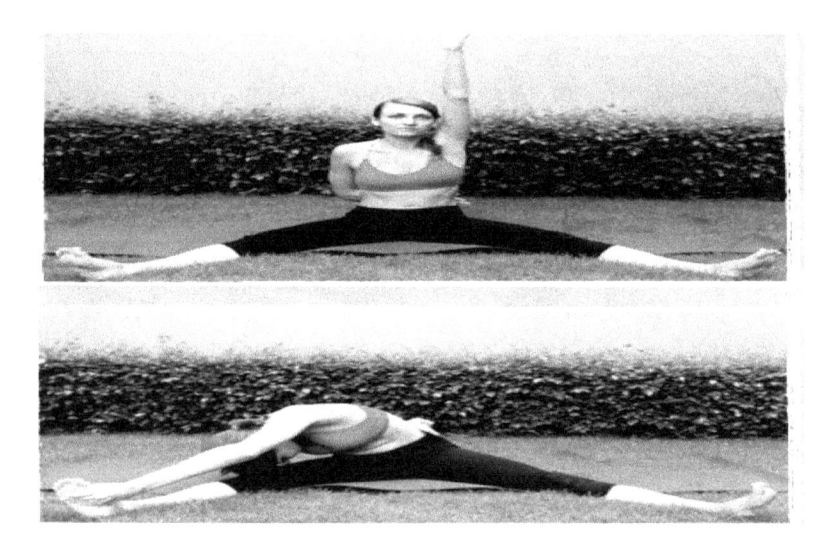

Twisted Pose I

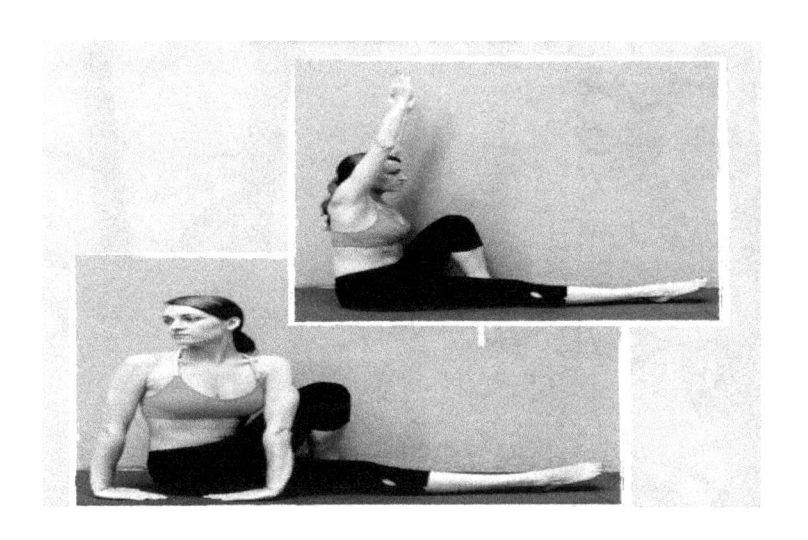

Twisted Pose II

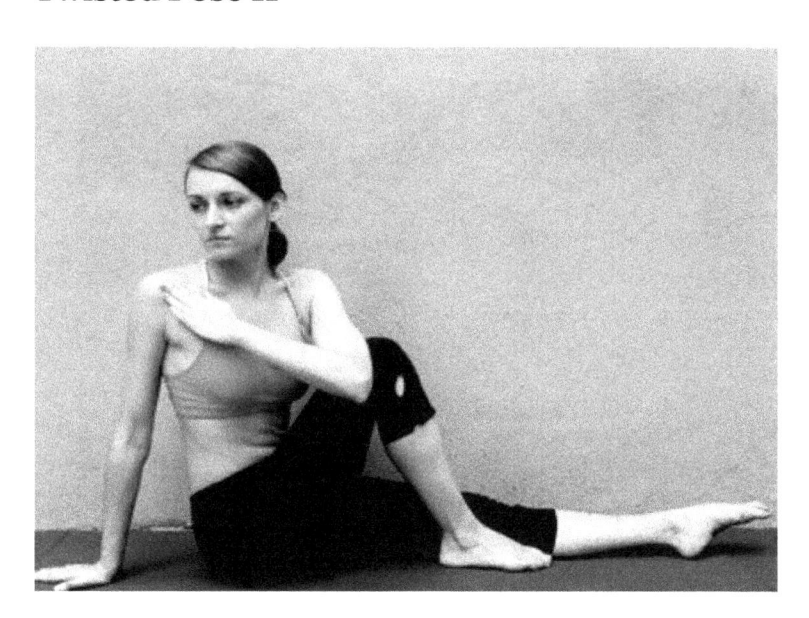

Sitting Half Boat Pose

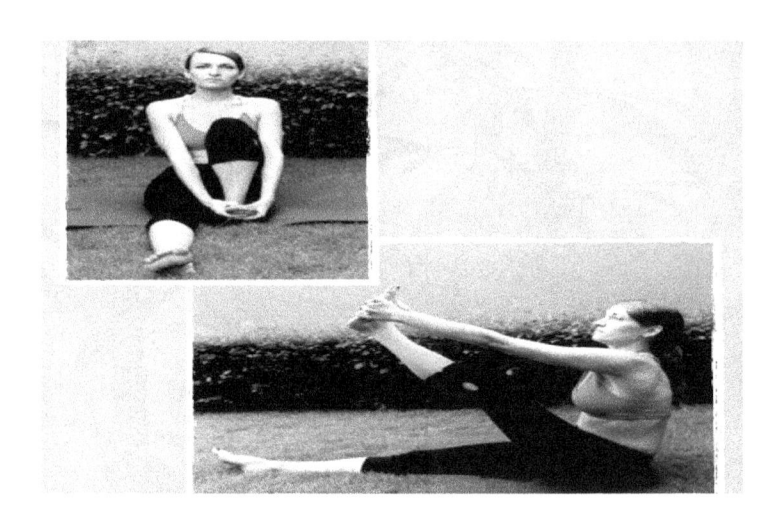

Twisted Forward Stretch

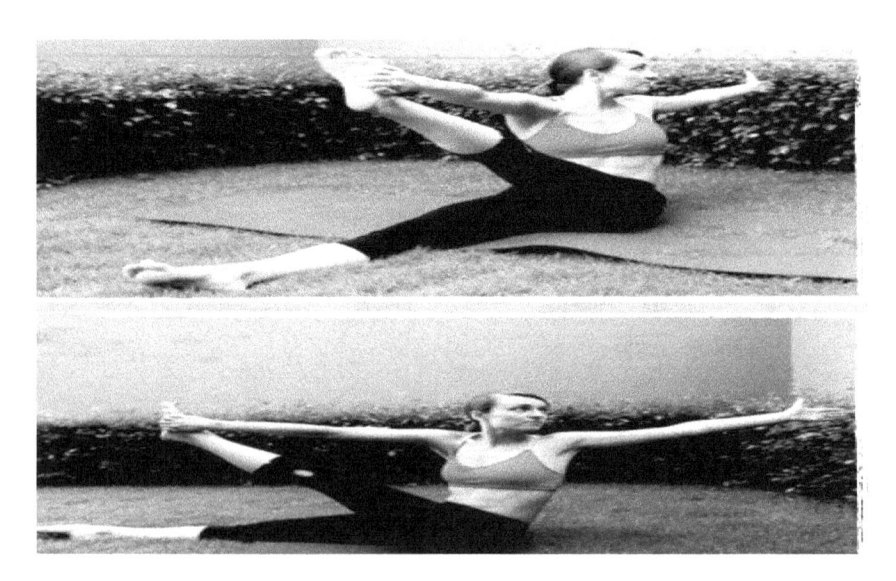

Hip Rocking Pose

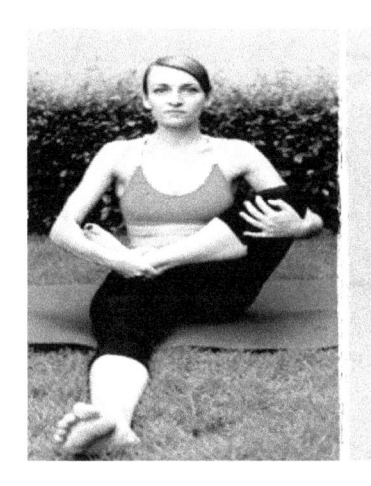

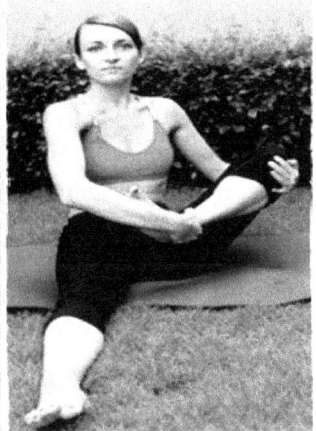

Butterfly Pose

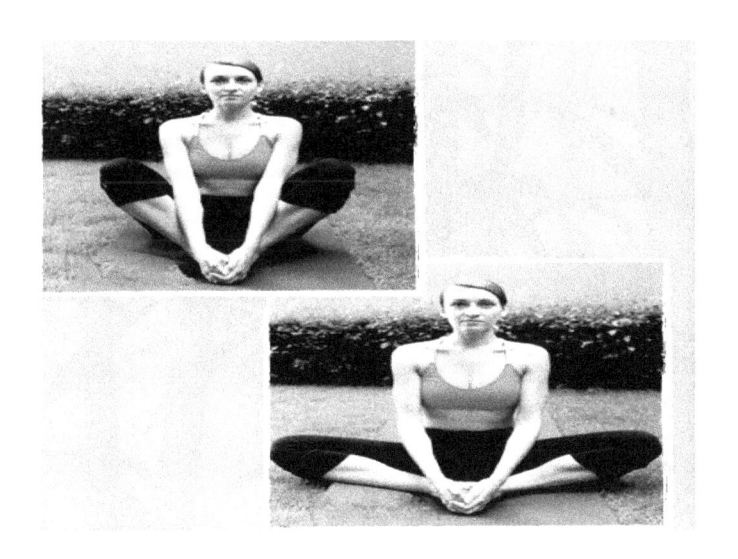

Cobbler's Pose

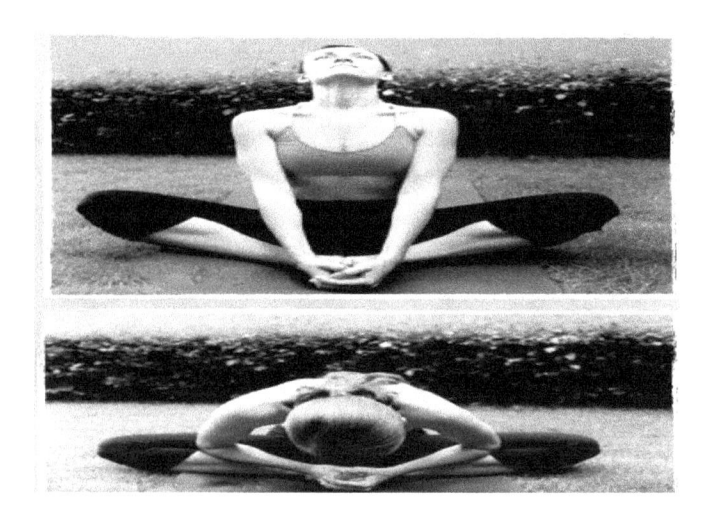

Knees Poses

Child's Pose

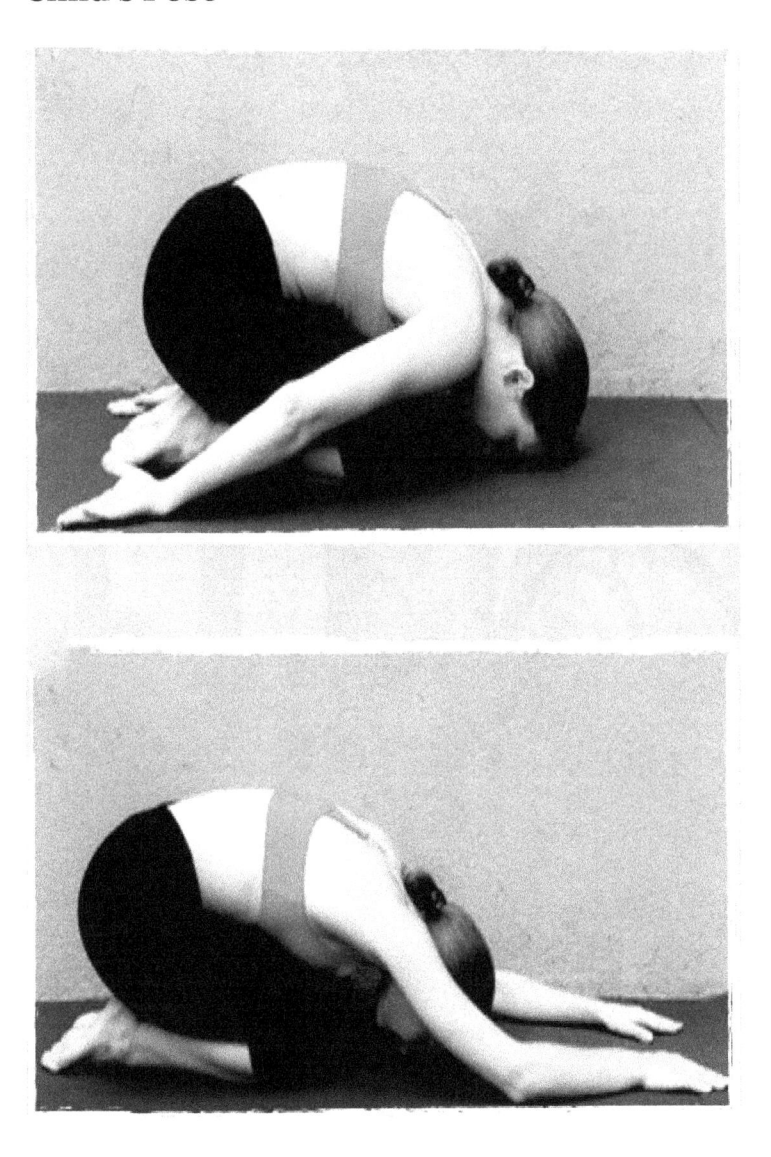

Cat Stretch

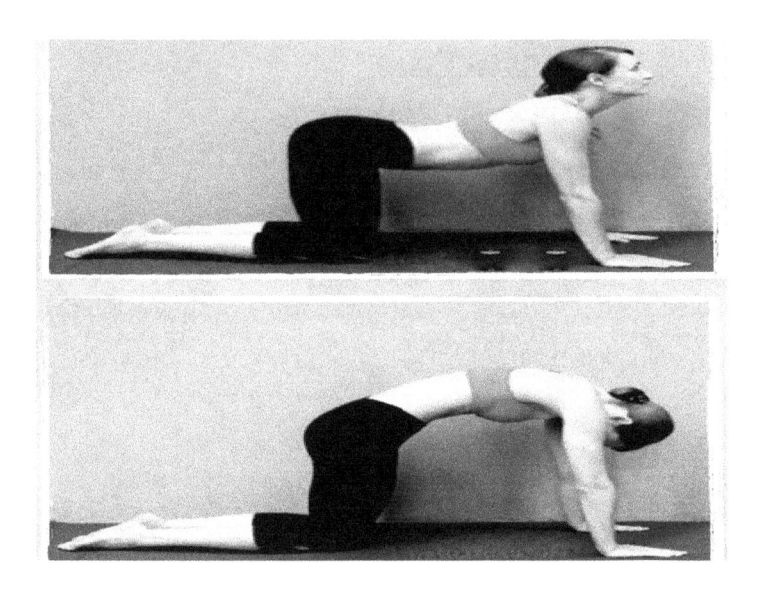

Alternate Leg-Hand Balance

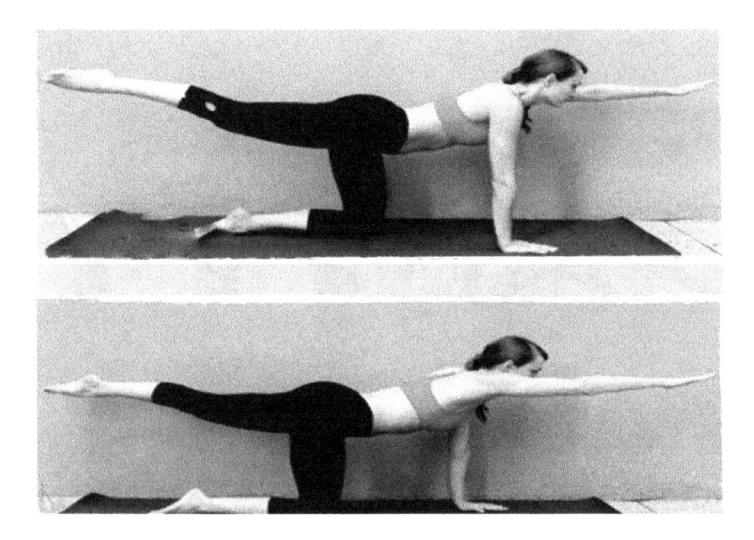

Tiger Pose

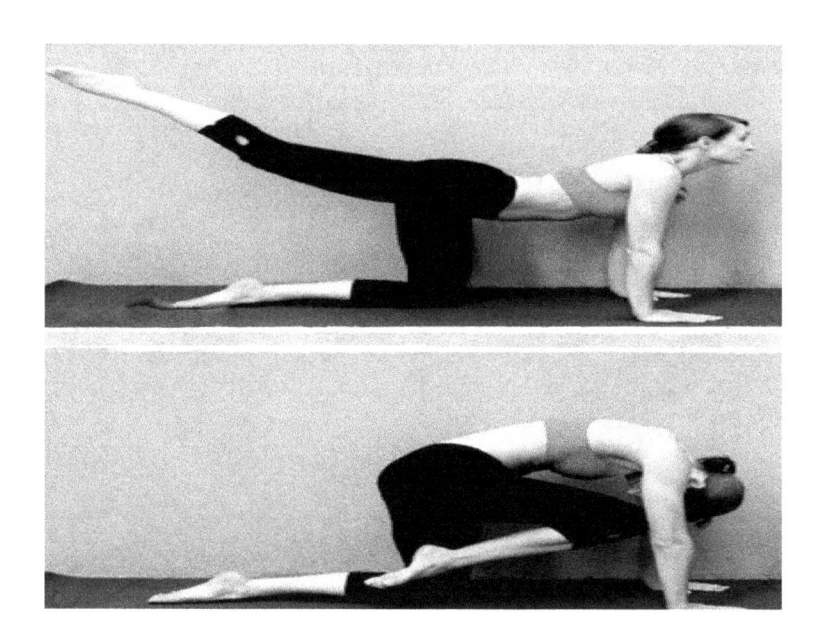

Downward Facing Dog

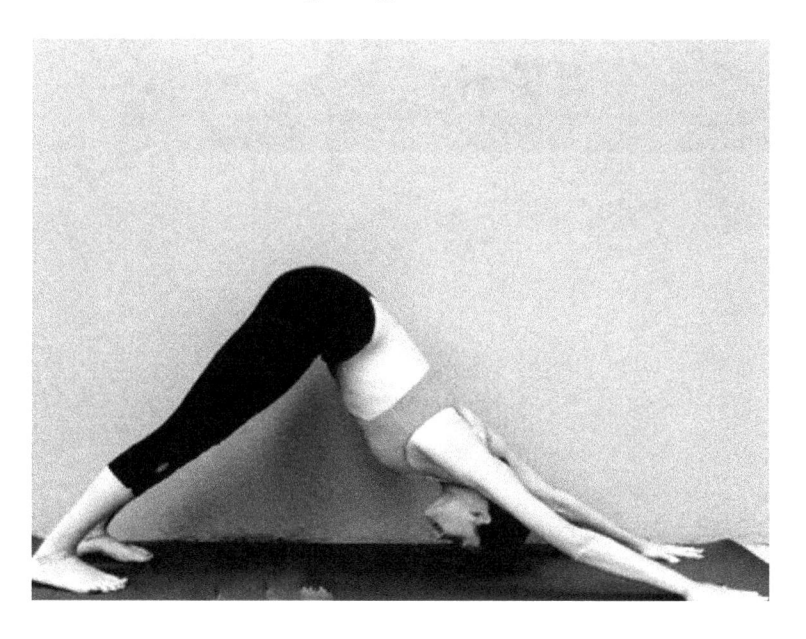

Raised Leg Downward Facing Dog

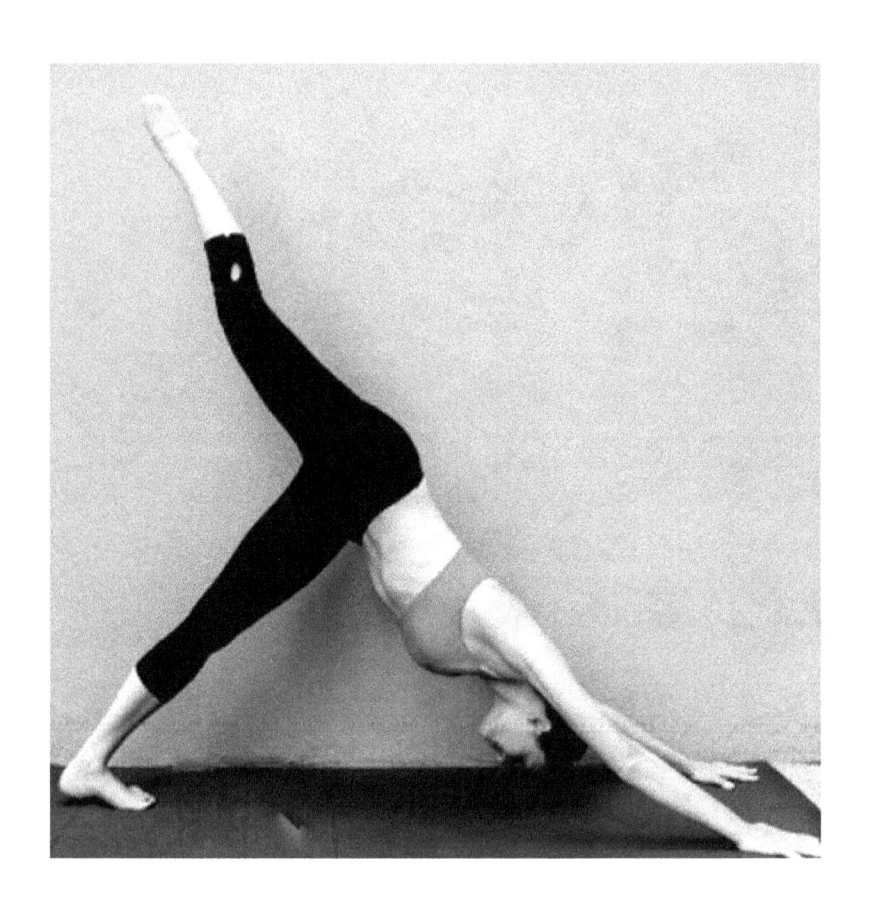

Closing Poses & Mudras

Gyana Mudra

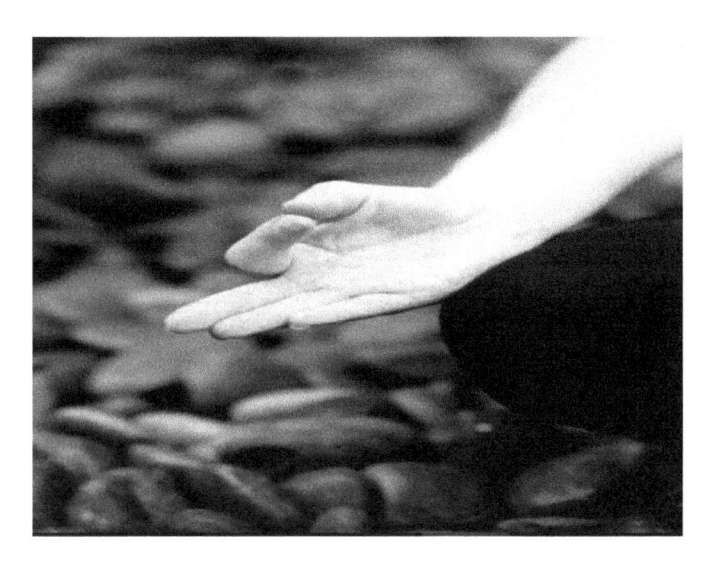

Surya Mudra

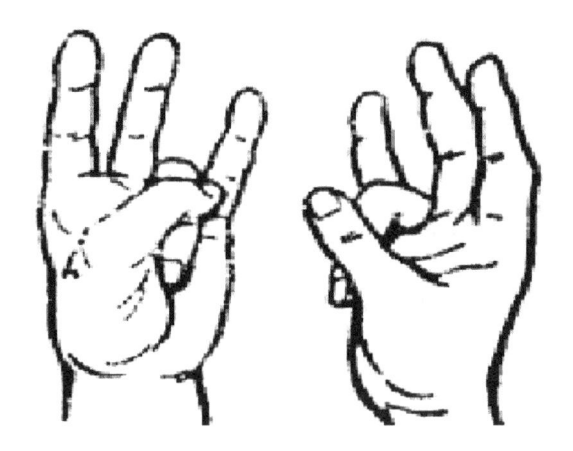

Palming

Mountain Pose

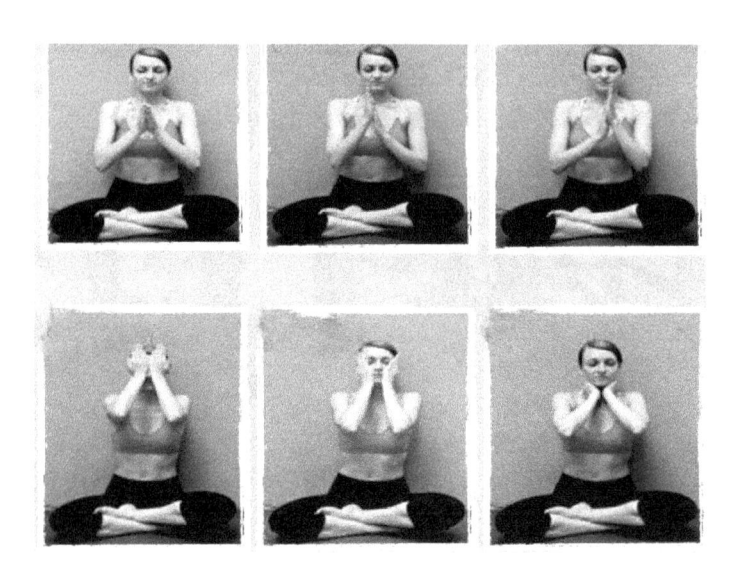

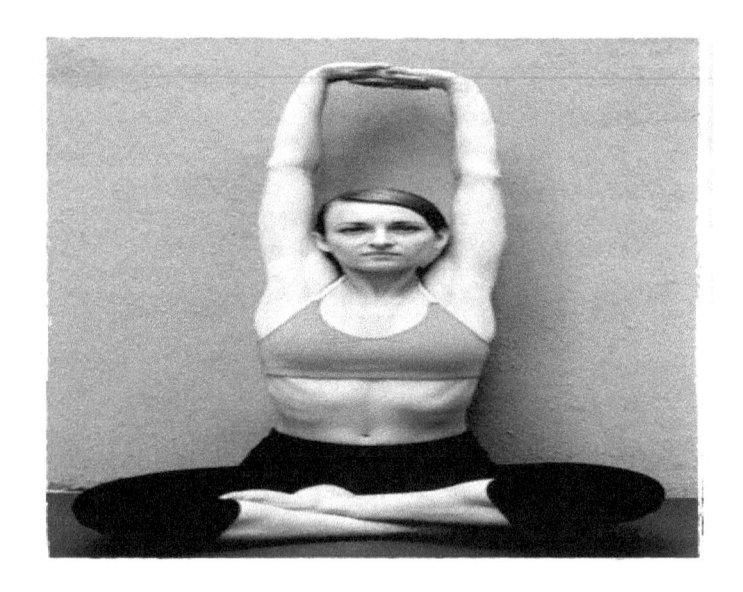

Side Mountain Pose

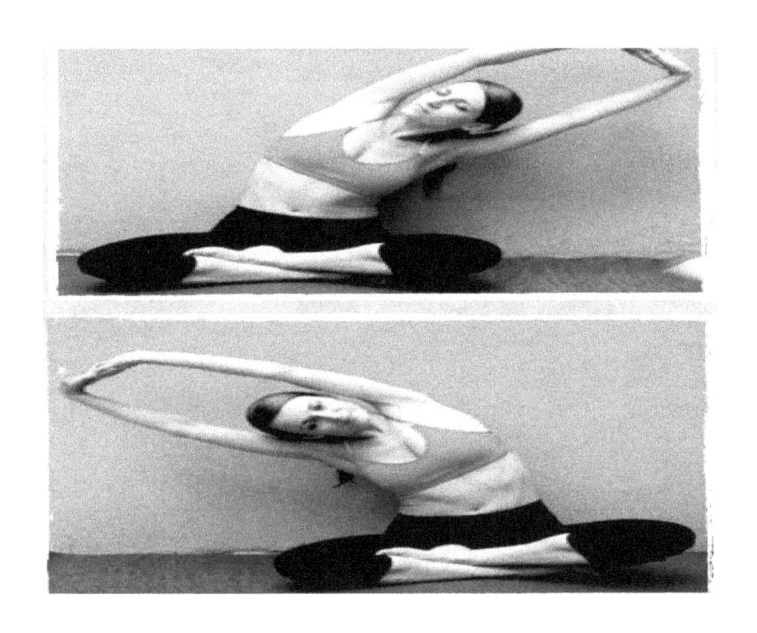

Surrender Pose

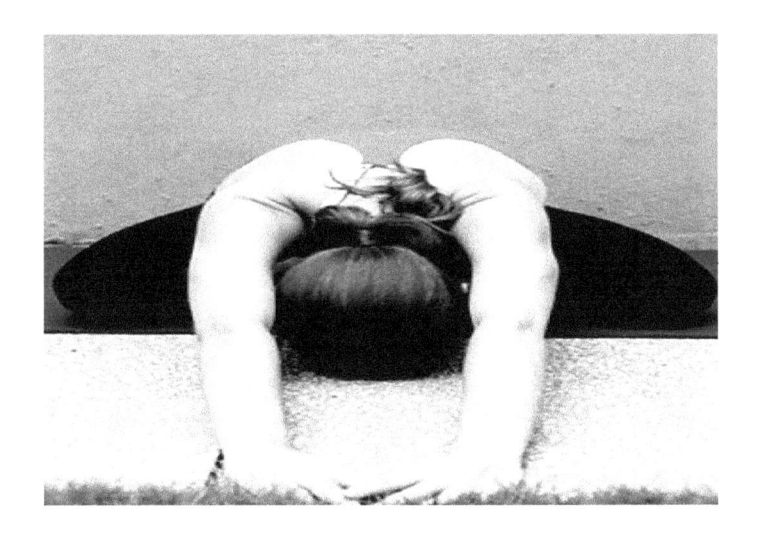

BASIC YOGA ROUTINES

Sun Salutations

Prayer pose

Instructions:

- stand upright,
- place your feet and hands flat on your chest — usually breathe

Standing Arch

Instructions:

- inhale and lift your two arms above your head
- bend your shoulders, arms and upper trunk slightly backward,
- lookup

Forward bend

Instructions:

- exhale and bend forward from the hips
- touch the floor with your fingers or palm of the hands
- Move your forehead as close to your knees as you can so you don't strain

Half cobra pose

Instructions:

- ❖ place your palms on the floor next to the feet, keep the arms straight
- ❖ breathe in and bring your left leg back
- ❖ drop your left knee on the floor and curve your right knee
- ❖ In the final pose, the left foot, two hands, left knee, and toes bolster the body.
- ❖ the back is somewhat angled, and the head looks ahead
- ❖ look upwards

Plank pose

Directions:

❖ Hold your breath and put your right leg back from Half Cobra, patch your knees and hands.

❖ drop the hips until the body frames a straight line from the highest point of your head to your heels

❖ center the look around the fixed point in front

Ashtanga positioning

Directions:

- ❖ breathe out and from Plank Pose
- ❖ bring down your knees, chest, and jaw on the floor; the feet will come up on to the toes

- In the final position, just the toes, knees, chest, hands and jaw (8 pieces of the body) should contact the floor
- the bottom, chips, and guts ought to be raised

Cobra pose

Directions:

- breathe in, keep your hands next to your chest and slide the chest forward
- raise first the head, the shoulders, at that point, fixing the elbows
- curve into the Cobra Pose
- this will bring down the hips and the bum to the floor
- bend the head back and look upward

Downward facing dog

Directions:

- Hold your breath, lift the hands and put down the head between the arms so that the back and the legs form the triangle on separate sides
- keep the knees and hands straight
- push the heels and head towards the floor

One leg forward curve

Directions:

- Stand upright with your legs together.

- Step forward with your left leg, Stand upright with your legs together.
- Turn your right foot to 45 degrees.
- unite your the two palms despite your good faith, interlock the fingers and spot your palms on your lower back
- Inhale, lift your head, extend your chest and look up the exhale bend, bring your forehead to the knee while holding both legs straight for five breaths
- lift your head to the starting position.
- Repeat on the right side

Precautions:

People with weak heart and low back issues should not practice this posture.

Benefits:

- opening hip and shoulders joints
- stretching the lower back
- contracting abdominal muscles helps to burn the fat in this area
- strengthening the legs

Triangle pose

Instructions:

- stand upright with no space between the legs

- Move forward with your left leg, raise your right foot at an angle of 45 degrees
- inhale, extend your arms horizontally on the shoulder level so that they are in one straight line
- exhale, lean to the left, bring your left hand down to your left foot and your right hand upwards
- keep your knees straight and your arms straight
- look up to your left hand in the final position and maintain the pose for five breaths
- Upon inhaling, return to the upright position with arms in a straight line
- exhale, release the hands on both sides of your body
- Redo this on the right side

Precautions: None

Benefits:

- toning the muscles on the side of the trunk, the waist and the back of the legs

- improving digestion

- helping to reduce waistline fat

One hand backbend

Instructions:

- stand straight with legs closed
- Step forward with your left leg, first rotate your right foot at a 45-degree angle
- inhale, stretch your arms out to the sides at shoulder level so that they are in a straight line
- exhale, lean your upper body back, raising your left hand, and your right-hand stays on your thigh
- keep your knees straight
- Look at the end of the left hand and hold the position for 5 seconds, return to the starting position with the arms in a straight line, exhale and drop your hands to the sides of the body.
- repeat on the right side Precautions: Make sure that you are tilting to the back and releasing the pose very slowly; otherwise you might feel dizzy

Benefits:

- toning the muscles on the side of the trunk, the waist and the back of the legs
- improving digestion

❖ helping to reduce waistline fat

Revolved triangle pose

Instructions:

❖ stand upstanding, ensuring the feet are more than shoulder-width separated

❖ turn the left foot to one side

❖ breathe in, raise the arms sideways to the shoulder level

❖ breathe out, curve the storage compartment to one side, twist advance and welcome your correct hand on the external side of the left foot and the left hand up, extended vertically with the goal that the two arms are framing a straight line

❖ gaze toward the left hand, keep your knees straight

❖ hold the final position for five breaths, adjusting the body and feeling the curve and stretch of the back

❖ breathe in, lift your hands to bear level

❖ breathe out, come back to the inside forward position

❖ repeat on the other side

Option:

If you can't place your hand on the outer side of the foot, you could place your palm on your ankle or calf - the most important is to keep the knees straight

Precautions

People suffering from back conditions shouldn't practice this posture

Precautions

People suffering from back conditions shouldn't practice this posture

Benefits:

❖ toning up the thigh, calf, hip and hamstring muscles

❖ reducing fat around the waist and hips

❖ strengthening and toning the arms

Side angle stretch

Instructions:

❖ Stand up with feet wider than a single shoulder width

❖ turn the left foot to one side

❖ breathe in, twist your left knee and spot your left elbow on the thigh, lean forward, with the goal that you left thigh is corresponding to the floor

❖ breathe out, broaden your correct arm over the ear until you structure a straight line from the tips of your fingers to the toes

❖look to your right side and hold the position for five breaths stance for five breaths

❖ breathe in, discharge the right hand to the back

❖ breathe out, come back to the beginning position

❖ rehash on the opposite side

Safety measures:

Individuals with feeble heart and lower back issues ought not to rehearse this stance

Benefits:

toning up ankles, knees, and thighs

❖ reducing fat around the waist and hips

❖ toning the legs

Revolved side angle stretch

Instructions:

❖ stand erect with the feet broadly spread apart

❖ breathe in, turn the left foot to one side

❖ breathe out, twist your left knee, twist forward, turn your trunk, unite your palms and spot your correct elbow on the external side of your left knee

❖ extend your chest up

❖ hold this posture for five breaths

❖ breathe in, discharge the hands to the front

❖ breathe out, come back to the beginning position

❖ rehash on the opposite side

Safety measures:

Individuals experiencing genuine back conditions and feeble knees shouldn't practice this stance Benefits:

❖ improving processing by contracting stomach organs

❖ the blood is flowing admirably around the stomach organs and the spinal section, and they are accordingly revived

❖ assisting with expelling waste issue from the colon without strain

Chest expand

Instructions:

❖ Stand upright with the feet widely spread apart

❖ inhale, lift both hands and tilt to the back

❖ extend the chest and hold it for a few seconds

❖ exhale, drop the hands and return to the starting position

Precautions:

People with low heart and back issues should not exercise this role.

Benefits:

❖ stretching arms and spine

❖ helping in deep breathing

❖ toning abdominal muscles

❖ strengthening the lower back, calves, and buttocks

Wide leg forward bend I

Instructions:

❖ stand erect with the feet generally spread separated

❖ breathe in, lift your two hands, tilt to the back and grow the chest

- breathe out, twist forward, place your palms on the floor and push your head towards the floor

- hold the stance for five breaths

- breathe in, gradually lift your head and hands up

- inhale out, discharge the hands and come back to the beginning position

Choice:

On the off chance that you can't contact your head to the floor, simply welcome your hands on the floor - don't strain, go just to the extent your body permits you

Safeguards:

Individuals with genuine neck/arm/shoulder issues ought not to rehearse this stance

Benefits:

- fortifying and thinning the arms and upper back

- extending the hamstrings

Wide leg forward twist

Instructions:

❖ From the Wide Leg Forward Bend I, place your left hand in the center of the floor and with inhaled twist your trunk and lift your right hand upwards

❖ two hands should shape a straight line, gaze upward

❖ hold the posture for five breaths

❖ breathe out, drop your left hand down to the floor

Precautions:

People with serious neck/arm/shoulder issues should not perform this pose

Benefits:

strengthening of arms, shoulders, chest, and upper back — toning of abdominal and lower back muscles

Warrior pose I

Instructions:

❖ Stand straight with your legs

❖ move forward with your left leg

❖ turn your right foot to 45 degrees

❖ place your palms on your hip, bend your hip so that the thigh is parallel to the floor

❖ inhale, lift your two hands, stretch your spine and look forward

❖ the bent knee does not reach past the ankle but should be in line with the heel.

❖ hold the posture for five long breaths

❖ breathe out and discharge your hands down, return to the beginning posture

❖ rehash on the correct side

Precautions:

Individuals with frail heart and lower back issues ought not to rehearse this stance

Warrior pose II

Instructions:

❖ stand upright with legs together

❖ step forward with left leg first, turn your right foot to 45 degrees

❖ Bend the left knee to connect thigh with the ground

❖ breathe in, stretch your hands sideways on the shoulder level and take a gander at your left palm

❖ your right knee stays straight

❖ the left knee ought not to reach out past the lower leg however ought to be following the heel

❖ hold the posture for five long breaths

❖ breathe out and discharge your hands down, return to the beginning posture

❖ rehash on the correct side

Precautions

People with weak heart and issues with the lower back need not perform this pose

Benefits:

❖leg muscles become shapely and more grounded

❖ carrying flexibility to the legs and back muscles and conditioning the stomach organs ❖ reinforcing the arms

Simple warrior present III

Directions:

❖ from Warrior Pose I, breathe out lower your left knee and twist the storage compartment forward

❖ lay the chest on the thigh and present your hands

❖ Keep your arms straight, and your hands close

❖ hold this situation for five long breaths

❖ breathe out, bring down your hands to the knee and raise while fixing your two legs

❖ go back to starting position

❖ repeat on the right side

Precautions:

People with a weak heart and lower back problems should not practice this posture

Benefits:

❖ contracting and toning stomach organs and making the leg muscles all the more shapely and solid

❖ assisting with disposing of fat in the stomach region and hips

❖ reinforcing the thighs

Easy half moon pose

Instructions:

❖ from Easy Warrior Pose III place your palms on the floor beside the feet, keep the arms straight

- inhale, raise your right leg, hold it parallel to the floor and straighten your left knee

- look down on the floor

- maintain the posture for five breaths

- breathe out, drop your correct leg on the floor and return to the beginning posture

- rehash on the opposite side

Safety measures:

Individuals with lower back issues ought not to rehearse this stance.

Benefits:

- reducing fat around the hips

- stretching the hamstrings, calves and thighs muscles

- toning the buttocks

Balancing Poses

Tree Pose

Directions:

- remain with the feet together and the arms by the sides

- consistent the body and appropriate the weight similarly on the two feet

- raise your left leg, twist the knee and spot the sole on the internal side of your correct thigh

- fix the eyes at one point and find the equalization

- breathe in, raise the arms over the head, unite the palms and stretch the arms, shoulders, and chest upward

- stretch the entire body through and through, without losing balance or moving the feet

- hold the situation for five breaths

- breathe out gradually discharge the arms and left leg down to the beginning position

- rehash on the opposite side

Precautionary measures:

Be cautious with the lower legs, warm it up before the training

Benefits:

- creating physical and mental equalization

- extending the abs and the digestion tracts, assisting with keeping the stomach muscles and nerves conditioned

❖ improving the stance

Standing Half Bow Balance

Guidelines:

❖ remain with the feet together and center around a fixed point

❖ breathe in, twist the left knee and handle the lower leg with the abandoned hand the body, lift the correct hand up

❖ keep the two knees together and keep up the equalization

❖ breathe out, gradually raise and stretch the right leg in reverse as high as agreeable

❖ arrive at upward and advance with the right arm

❖ center the look around your right hand

❖ hold the situation for five breaths

❖ breathe in, bring down the right arm to the side, bring down the left leg, uniting the knees

❖ Breathe out, discharge the left lower leg, and lower the foot to the floor, bring down the correct arm to the side.

❖ rehash on the opposite side

Precautions:

Individuals who experience the ill effects of a feeble heart, hypertension, back issues, hernia, colitis, peptic or duodenal ulcers or vertigo ought not to rehearse it

Benefits:

❖ reinforcing the back, shoulders, arms, hips, and legs

❖ building up a feeling of parity and coordination and improving focus

Standing Knee To Chest Balance

Directions:

❖ remain with the feet together and the arms by the sides

❖ breathe in, raise your left leg, seize the shin and bring the knee near the chest with toes pointing down

❖ stretch the entire body start to finish, without losing balance or moving the feet

❖ fix the eyes at one point and find the equalization

❖ hold the situation for five breaths

❖ breathe out gradually discharge the arms and left leg down to the beginning position

❖ rehash on the opposite side

Safety measures:

Be cautious with the lower legs, warm it up before the training.

Benefits:

❖ creating physical and mental parity

❖ extending the muscular strength and the digestion tracts, assisting with keeping the abs and nerves conditioned

❖ improving the stance and fortifying the arms

❖ animating processing

Standing Knee Side Balance

Guidelines:

❖ from the Standing Knee To Chest Balance, breathe in and carry your bowed knee to one side and your correct hand to the right side on the shoulder level

❖ stretch the entire body through and through, without losing balance or moving the feet

❖ fix the eyes at one point and find the equalization

- ❖ hold the situation for five breaths

- ❖ breathe out, gradually discharge the left leg to the front and drop the foot on the floor

- ❖ take the correct hand back to the side

- ❖ rehash on the opposite side

Safeguards:

Be cautious with the lower legs, warm it up before the training.

Benefits:

- ❖ creating physical and mental equalization

- ❖ extending the muscular strength and the digestive organs, assisting with keeping the abs and nerves conditioned

- ❖ improving the stance

- ❖ fortifying the arms and lower back

Falcon Pose

Guidelines

- ❖ remain with the feet together and the arms by the sides

- hold the left leg straight, twist the correct leg and curve it around the left leg

- the right thigh ought to be before the left thigh, and the highest point of the right foot should lay on the calf of the left leg

- twist the elbows and get them in front of the chest

- breathe in, curve the lower arms around one another with the left elbow staying beneath

- place the palms together to take after and eagle's mouth

- balance right now, breathe out, gradually twist the left knee and lower the body, keeping the back straight

- keep the eyes concentrated on the fixed point

- hold the final position for five breaths, at that point raise the body, and discharge the legs and arms

- rehash on the opposite side

Precautionary measures:

Individuals with tight knees ought to be cautious with this stance

Benefits:

- ❖ fortifying the muscles and relaxing the joints of the shoulders, arms, and legs

- ❖ It's useful for extending the upper back

- ❖ improving fixation

Seat Pose

Guidelines:

- ❖ remain with the feet together and the arms by the sides

- ❖ breathe in, raise the arms over the head

- ❖ breathe out, twist the knees and lower the storage compartment

- ❖ don't stoop forward, however, keep the chest as far back as could be allowed and inhale ordinarily

- ❖ keep your back straight and hold the posture for five breaths

- ❖ breathe in, fix the legs,

- ❖ breathe out, bring down the arms and return to standing posture

Precautionary measures:

Individuals experiencing severe back conditions ought to keep away from this stance

Benefits:

❖ expelling firmness in the shoulders

❖ the lower legs become stable, and the leg muscles grow equally

❖ the stomach is lifted, and this gives a delicate back rub to the heart

❖ the stomach organs and the back are conditioned, and the chest is reinforced by being completely extended

Pussyfoot Pose

Directions:

❖ remain with the feet together and the arms by the sides

❖ breathe in, raise on the toes and bring your hands upon the shoulder level

❖ breathe out, squat with the look concentrated on a fixed point

❖ raise the heels and equalization on the pussyfoots

❖ permit the knees to approach marginally with the goal that the thighs are corresponding to the floor

❖ place your palms on the thighs, fix your back and parity the entire body

❖ remain right now five breaths

❖ discharge the posture, drop your knees on the floor, and sit between your feet to loosen up

Precautions:

Individuals with sciatica slipped circle, lower leg or knee issues ought not to rehearse this asana

Benefits:

❖ fortifying the toes, lower legs, lower back, and thighs

❖ improving equalization and fixation

Sitting Poses

Simple Meditation Pose

Guidelines:

❖ sit with legs straight before the body

❖ twist the two legs and cross it before your body

❖ place the hands on the knees

- close your eyes

- keep the head, neck, and back upstanding and straight

- loosen up the entire body

- arms ought to be loose and not held straight

Safety measures:

Individuals with extreme knees issues ought not to be sitting right now excessively long

Benefits:

- this is the simplest and most agreeable reflective posture

- it encourages mental and physical parity without strain or torment

Half Lotus Pose

Directions:

- sit with legs straight before the body

- twist one leg and spot the sole within the contrary thigh

- turn the other leg and place the foot on the contrary thigh

❖ with no strain, attempt to put the upper heel as close as conceivable to the belly

❖ alter the position with the goal that it is agreeable

❖ place the hands on the knees and close your eyes

❖ keep the head, neck, and back upstanding and straight

❖ loosen up the entire body

❖ arms ought to be loose and not held straight

Safeguards:

Individuals experiencing sciatica or frail or harmed knees ought not to play out this stance

Benefits:

❖ permitting the body to be kept consistent for significant stretches, holding the storage compartment and head like a column with the legs as a firm establishment

❖ applying strain to the lower spine, which relaxingly affects the sensory system

❖ the breath turns out to be moderate, the intense pressure is diminished, and the pulse is decreased

❖ the typically massive blood flow of the legs is diverted to the stomach district animating the stomach related procedure.

Lotus Pose

Directions:

- sit with legs straight before the body

- twist the left knee and spot the left foot on the correct thigh

- bend the right knee and spot the right foot on the left thigh

- alter the posture with the goal that it is agreeable; the knees ought to be firmly on the floor

- place the hands on the knees and close your eyes

- keep the head, neck, and back upstanding and straight

- loosen up the entire body

- arms ought to be loose and not held straight

Safety measures:

Individuals with sciatica or sacral contaminations ought not to play out this stance

Benefits:

- it's a sound situation to sit in, particularly for those experiencing varicose veins, drained and hurting muscles or fluid maintenance in the legs

❖ it expands the efficiency of the whole stomach related framework, soothing stomach diseases, for example, hyperacidity and peptic ulcer

❖ you can rehearse Vajrasana straightforwardly after dinners for in any event 5 minutes to improve the stomach related capacity

Jolt Pose I

Guidelines:

❖ stoop on the floor with the knees near one another

❖ unite the enormous toes and separate the heels

❖ Bring down the backside onto within the surface of the feet with the impact points contacting the sides of the hips.

❖ Place your hands on the hips, your palms down

❖ the back and head ought to be straight yet not tense

❖ close the eyes, loosen up the arms and the entire body

Choice:

If there is a torment in the thighs or lower legs, the knees might be isolated while keeping up the stance. You can likewise put the cushion underneath your backside and sit on it.

Precautionary measures:

Be cautious with your lower legs and knees

Benefits:

❖ modifying the flow of blood and apprehensive driving forces into the pelvic area and fortifying the pelvic muscles

❖ expanding the efficiency of the whole stomach related

Two Legs Forward Bend I

Instructions:

❖ sit down on the floor with your legs oustretched and spread apart as far as possible

❖ breathe in, lift two hands over the head

❖ breathe out, twist forward and seize your left toe with your left hand and right toe with your right hand

❖ attempt to carry your brow to the floor in the middle of the knees, keep the two knees straight

❖ hold the posture for five breaths

❖ breathe in, lift your two hands and head up

❖ breathe out, discharge two hands on the floor alongside the thighs

Safety measures:

Individuals experiencing slipped plate, sciatica or hernia ought not to rehearse this stance

Benefits:

❖ extending hamstring muscles and expanding flexibility in the hip joints and spine

❖ conditioning and kneading the whole stomach and pelvic district

❖ expelling overabundance weight in the stomach region and invigorating flow to the nerves and muscles of the spine

Two Legs Forward Bend II

Instructions:

❖ plunk down on the floor with your legs outstretched, feet together

❖ breathe in, lift your two hands over the head

❖ breathe out twist forward, slide the hands down the legs and seize your feet (elective: lower legs, calves)

❖ bring your head as close as conceivable to the knees, keeping your knees straight

❖ hold the posture for five breaths

❖ breathe in, lift two hands up

❖ breathe out, discharge two hands on the floor by the thighs

Precautionary measures:

Individuals experiencing slipped circle, sciatica, or hernia ought not to rehearse this asana Benefits:

❖ extending hamstring muscles and expanding flexibility in the hip joints and spine

❖ conditioning and rubbing the whole stomach and pelvic locale

❖ evacuating abundance weight in the stomach region and animating course to the nerves and muscles of the spine

Contorted Pose I

Directions:

❖ plunk down on the floor with your legs outstretched, feet together

- ❖ twist the left knee and spot the foot on the floor

- ❖ breathe in, lift your two hands over the head

- ❖ breathe out, turn the storage compartment to the correct side and place the right palm behind the right butt cheek, and the left palm beside the right thigh, with the fingers highlighting one another

- ❖ curve the head and trunk as far to one side as is open to, utilizing the arms as switches, while keeping the spine upstanding and straight

- ❖ the rear end ought to stay on the floor; the correct elbow may twist a bit, however, attempt to keep it straight

- ❖ investigate the correct shoulder beyond what many would consider possible without stressing, feel the curve in the lower back

- ❖ hold the final position for five breaths

- ❖ inhale, straighten your head and raise both hands above the head, re-center the trunk

- ❖ exhale, release the hands, repeat on the other side

Precautions:

People with back complaints should be careful with this posture

Benefits:

❖ stretching the spine, loosening the vertebrae and toning the nerves

❖ alleviating backache, neck pain lumbago and mild forms of sciatica

Twisted Pose II

Instructions:

❖ sit down on the floor with your legs outstretched, feet together

❖ twist the right knee and spot the foot on the floor

❖ breathe in, lift your two hands over the head

❖ breathe out, turn the storage compartment to the right side and spot the right palm behind the right butt cheek, and the left palm on the right shoulder, the left elbow is pushing on the right knee

❖ curve the head and trunk as far to the right as is open to, utilizing the arms as switches, while keeping the spine upright and straight

❖ the rear end ought to stay on the floor

❖ investigate the right shoulder quite far without stressing, feel the wind in the lower back

❖ hold the final position for five breaths

❖ inhale, straighten your head and raise both hands above the head, re-center the trunk

❖ exhale, release the hands, repeat on the other side

Precautions:

People with back complaints should be careful with this posture

Benefits:

❖ stretching the spine, loosening the vertebrae and toning the nerves

❖ alleviating backache, neck pain lumbago and mild forms of sciatica

Sitting Half Boat Pose

Instructions:

❖ sit down on the floor with your legs outstretched, feet together

❖ Inhale, bend the left knee, raise the left foot (alternative: leg, heel, calf).

❖ keep the back and knee straight and try to bring your leg as close as possible to the forehead

❖ gaze at the big toe and hold the pose for five breaths

❖ exhale, slowly release the leg on the floor

❖ repeat on the other side

Precautions:

People with back complaints or a displaced coccyx should not practice this pose.

Benefits:

❖ rendering the hamstring muscles and improving flexibility of hip joints

❖ toning abdominal muscles

❖ strengthening arms and spine muscles

Twisted Forward Stretch

Instructions:

❖ from the Sitting, Half Boat Pose inhale and grab hold the outer side of your left foot (option: ankle, heel, calf) with your right hand

❖ twist the trunk towards the left side, extend the left arm to the back at the shoulder level

❖ turn the head to the back and gaze over the left shoulder at your left palm

❖ keep your knees and back straight

❖ hold the pose for five breaths

❖ exhale, straighten your head and trunk, release your left hand and bring the left leg down on the floor

❖ repeat on the other side

Precautions:

People with back complaints or a displaced coccyx should not practice this asana

Benefits:

❖ rendering the hamstring muscles and improving flexibility of hip joints

❖ toning abdominal muscles

❖ strengthening arms and spine muscles

❖ a gentle twist of the lower back is strengthening lower back muscles

Hip Rocking Pose

Instructions:

❖ sit down on the floor with the legs outstretched, feet together

❖ Inhale, bend the left leg, raise the left knee and ankle and bring the hip sideways

❖ straighten your back, and start rocking the hip to the left and right (movement reminds rocking the baby)

❖ swing the leg for five breaths

❖ slowly release the leg on the floor

❖ repeat on the other side

Precautions:

People with back complaints or a displaced coccyx should not practice this pose.

Benefits:

❖ opening and releasing tension in the hip

❖ improving flexibility of the hip joints

❖ toning abdominal muscles

❖ strengthening the spine

Butterfly Pose

Instructions:

- ❖ plunk down on the floor with the legs outstretched, feet together

- ❖ Breathe in, pull in your feet, and spot the bottoms of the feet together, as close as conceivable to your pelvis, let the knees drop out to the sides.

- ❖ ricochet the knees delicately (like a butterfly flapping it's wings)

- ❖ breath typically and continue bobbing the knees for the span of 5 breaths

- ❖ discharge the legs and return to the beginning position

Insurances:

Individuals with sciatica or knee issues ought not to rehearse this posture.

Benefits:

- ❖ improving the flexibility in the crotch and hips district

- ❖ easing the inward thigh muscles strain

- ❖ expelling tiredness from extended periods of strolling or standing

- ❖ setting up the legs for other thoughtful stances

Shoemaker's Pose

Directions:

❖ plunk down on the floor with the legs outstretched, feet together

❖ Breathe in, pull in your feet, and spot the bottoms of the feet together, as close as conceivable to your pelvis, let the knees drop out to the sides. Keep the spinal line and the neck straight.

❖ breathe in, handle your feet, raise your head and curve to the back

❖ breathe out, twist forward, bringing your brow down to the enormous toes

❖ press the elbows against the thighs, carrying them closer to the floor

❖ hold the posture for five breaths

❖ breathe in, raise the head and trunk up

❖ Breathe out, come back to the beginning posture
Precautions: People with sciatica or knee issues ought not to rehearse this posture.

Benefits:

❖ improving the flexibility in the crotch and hips area

- ❖ diminishing the internal thigh muscles pressure

- ❖ relieving the lower stomach organs and helping the excretory framework expel squander from the body

Knees Poses

Child's Pose

Instructions:

- ❖ kneel on the floor, touch your big toes together and sit in between your heels, (you can separate the knees)

- ❖ inhale, look up and stretch the back

- ❖ exhale, bend forward bringing the chest to the thighs and forehead on the floor

- ❖ bring your hands to the back and lay them down on the floor next to the hips (option: you can bring the hands in the front of the body as far as you can reach)

- ❖ hold this position for five long breaths, relax

- ❖ inhale, raise your head and trunk up

- ❖ exhale, release the pose

Precautions:

People having diarrhea or knee injury should avoid this pose.

Benefits:

- gently stretching the hips, thighs, and ankles

- it's a restorative posture, it helps you relax, calm down, relieves stress and fatigue

- Restoring body strength and relieving back, shoulders and chest stress

- practice it after Sun Salutations and in between sequences

Cat Stretch

Instructions:

- sit down in Thunderbolt Pose, raise the buttocks and stand on the knees

- lean forward and place the hands flat on the floor beneath the shoulders with the fingers facing forward

- the hands should be in line with the knees; the arms and thighs should be perpendicular to the floor

- do not bend the arms at the elbows, keep the arms and thighs vertical throughout

- inhale, raise the head and depress the spine

- exhale, arch your back, bring the chin to the chest

- repeat this movement for ten times

Precautions:

Be careful with your knees and neck

Benefits:

- improving the flexibility of the neck, shoulders, and spine

- toning the digestive system muscles

- massaging to the spine and abdominal organs

Alternate Leg-Hand Balance

Instructions:

- sit down in Thunderbolt Pose, raise the buttocks and stand on the knees

- lean forward and place the hands flat on the floor beneath the shoulders with the fingers facing forward

- the hands should be in line with the knees; the arms and thighs should be perpendicular to the floor

- Inhale, lift left and right leg parallel to the floor

- balance the body, look forward

- hold the pose for five breaths

- exhale, release the left hand and right leg

- repeat on the other side

Precautions:

People with knees or lower back problems should avoid this practice.

Benefits:

❖ improving the flexibility of the spine and lower back

❖ toning and shaping the abdominal muscles

❖ slimming effect on thighs, buttocks, and arms

Tiger Pose

Instructions:

❖ expect the beginning situation for Cat Stretch and look forward

❖ breathe in, discourage the back, fix the left leg, stretch it up to the back and look upwards

❖ breathe out, twist the left knee and swing the leg forward, bring the knee as close as conceivable to the brow

❖ rehash the development multiple times

❖ practice on the opposite side

Precautionary measures:

Individuals with later or ceaseless wounds of the back, hips or knees ought to dodge this stance

Benefits:

❖ practicing and relaxing the back by twisting it then again in the two headings, conditioning the spinal nerves

❖ soothing sciatica and relaxing up the legs and hip joints

❖ extending the abs,

❖ advancing assimilation and animating blood flow

❖ lessening weight from the hips and thighs

Downward Facing Dog

Instructions:

❖ Assume the Cat Stretch starting spot, and look ahead.

❖ Inhale, lift your hips and lower your head between your arms to form two sides of the triangle.

❖ keep the knees and hands straight, gaze on the floor

❖ push the heels and head towards the floor

❖ hold the pose for five breaths

❖ release the pose, relax in the Child's Pose

Precautions:

People with diarrhea, headache, high blood pressure or carpal tunnel syndrome should not practice this posture

Benefits:

❖ calming the brain and relieving stress

❖ energizing the body

❖ stretching the arms, shoulders, hamstrings, and calfs

❖ slimming effect on arms and legs

❖ improving digestion, relieving headache, insomnia, back pain, and fatigue

Raised Leg Downward Facing Dog

Instructions:

❖ from the Downward Facing Dog inhale, raise your left leg, as high as possible, keep it straight ❖ press the palms evenly into the floor, keep the elbows straight and move the chest towards the right thigh

❖ push the right heel towards the floor, look down

❖ hold the posture for five breaths

- exhale, release the left leg to Downward Facing Dog and repeat on the other side

Precautions:

People with high blood pressure, diarrhea, headache, or back condition, especially slipped discs should not practice this asana.

Benefits:

- strengthening the nerves and muscles in the limbs and back
- stretching, toning and shaping leg muscles and ligaments
- slimming effect on arms and legs ❖ improving digestion, relieving headache, insomnia, back pain, and fatigue

Closing Poses & Mudras

Gyana Mudra

Instructions

- Place the thumb tip on the index fingertip while the other fingers are relaxed and joined together

- assume this mudra with both hands and place them on the knees or thighs thigh, relax Benefits:

- enhancing mental capabilities, sharpening the memory, mental concentration

- beneficial for those suffering from insomnia, depression, anxiety

- increasing the smooth glow or blood supply and circulation in the brain to help energize the neurons for instant action

- it's a necessary psycho-neural finger lock which makes meditation more powerful

- the palms and fingers have many nerve root endings that continuously emit energy; when the index finger touches the thumb, a circuit is formed, which allows the energy that would usually dissipate into the environment to travel back through the body and up to the brain.

Mudra is the science of hand and finger postures. It can help to cure bodily ailments. It affects the body's energetic system and the flow of life energy within it.

Surya Mudra

Instructions:

- place the tip of the ring finger on the base of the thumb

- bring gentle pressure of the thumb upon ring finger.

- this amounts to suppression of element earth (residing in the ring finger) by element fire (living in the thumb)

Benefits:

- stimulating the thyroid gland improving metabolism

- helping to fight obesity, progressive weight-gain

- curing loss of appetite, indigestion, and constipation

- the increasing Fire element in the body responsible for burning fat

- it can also cure low body-temperature, the coldness of skin, body, limbs, hands, feet, etc.

- curing mental heaviness

Palming

Instructions

- sit down in a meditative pose (Easy Meditation Pose, Half Lotus Pose or Lotus Pose) ❖ close your eyes, breathe normally, relax

- while keeping your eyes closed, bring your palms together and start rubbing the palms until they feel warm

- slowly palm your eyes, avoid applying pressure on the eyeballs
- keep your eyes covered for few seconds
- release the hands, rub the palms one more time
- palm the cheeks, hold it for few seconds
- free the hands, rub the palms one more time
- palm the neck, hold it for few seconds
- release the hands, keep your eyes closed for few more seconds, then slowly open the eyes and release the meditative pose

Benefits:

- relaxing and revitalizing the eye, face and neck muscles
- stimulating the liquid that flows between the cornea and the lens of the eye
- aiding the correction of defective vision
- bringing relaxation to the entire body
- perfect practice for the beginning and end of a Yoga session

Mountain Pose

Directions:

❖ plunk down in any thoughtful pose (Easy Meditation Pose, Half Lotus Pose or Lotus Pose)

❖ breathe in, lift your two hands over the head, interlock the fingers, palms confronting upwards

❖ Stretch out your entire body.

❖ Look ahead for a few moments and keep the stretch

❖ breathe out, discharge the hands on the floor Precautions: People experiencing sciatica or powerless or harmed knees ought not to play out this stance

Benefits:

❖ fortifying the muscular strength, stomach related framework and spine muscles

❖ soothing pressure from the lower back

❖ loosening up the entire body

Side Mountain Pose

Directions

❖ plunk down in any thoughtful pose (Easy Meditation Pose, Half Lotus Pose or Lotus Pose)

❖ breathe in, lift your two hands over the head, interlock the fingers, palms confronting upwards

- ❖ stretch your entire body up

- ❖ breathe out, twist the storage compartment and outstretched arms to one side

- ❖ look to one side and up, hold the pose for few moments

- ❖ Breathe in, focus the hands and trunk and rehash on the opposite side

Precautions: People experiencing sciatica, feeble or harmed knees, or after late stomach medical procedure ought not to play out this stance.

Benefits:

- ❖ reinforcing the muscular strength, stomach related framework and spine muscles

- ❖ tenderly extending and cutting the abdomen

- ❖ easing strain from the lower back

- ❖ loosening up the entire body

Surrender Pose

Directions:

❖ plunk down in any thoughtful pose (Easy Meditation Pose, Half Lotus Pose or Lotus Pose) ❖ breathe in, lift your two hands over the head, interlock the fingers, palms confronting upwards

❖ stretch your entire body up

❖ breathe out, twist your trunk advance and acquire the outstretched hands front on the floor ❖ attempt to contact the brow to the floor and stretch the spine

❖ hold the pose for few moments, inhale regularly

❖ breathe in, gradually lift the storage compartment and hands, return to the sitting pose

❖ breathe out, discharge the hands and thoughtful pose

Safety measures:

Individuals experiencing sciatica or frail or harmed knees ought not to play out this stance

Benefits:

❖ reinforcing the muscular strength, stomach related framework and spine muscles

❖ pressure on the abdominal organs stimulates digestion

❖ relieving tension from the lower back and arms

❖ relaxing the whole body

YOGA DIET

Nutrition is the entirety of the procedure by which the living life form gets and uses the materials vital for endurance, development, and fix of destroyed tissues. Nourishment is the wellspring of the fuel, which is changed over by the metabolic procedure of the body into the vitality for crucial exercises. Calorimetry manages the estimation of vitality prerequisites of the body under different physiologic conditions and of the fuel estimations of the nourishment that supply this vitality. This unit of energy contained in nourishments, just as that engaged with metabolic exercises, is frequently communicated as a unit of warmth, the calorie. The worldwide unit of energy is the joule.

The burning of a staple within sight of oxygen brings about the creation of warmth. The measure of heat along these lines delivered can be estimated in a bomb calorimeter. By this method, the calorie estimation of a staple can be resolved. The warmth produced by the body throughout the digestion of groceries keeps up the internal heat level. Warm-blooded creatures, for example, winged animals and well-evolved creatures, have heat-controlling components that either increment that creation or transmit or, in any case, disseminate overabundance heat, contingent upon the temperature of their outer condition.

The entirety of the vitality delivered in the body is at last dispersed as warmth. Estimation of the original warmth creation of a creature is an approach to evaluate is vitality consumption. There are two strategies for achieving this:

A. Direct Calorimetry

B. Indirect Calorimetry

By measuring gas exchange and determining the respiratory quotient(RO) energy metabolism studies are considerably simplified and thus rendered applicable to field studies and to clinical analysis. The ratio of the amount of CO_2 removed to the amount of oxygen used in oxidation is the respiratory quotient. The RQ for carbohydrate is 1; for fats 0.7 and proteins 0.8. The total heat production or energy expenditure of the body is the sum of that required merely to maintain life (basal metabolism), together with which additional energy may be expanded for any other activities. The lowest level of energy production constant with life is the basal metabolic rate. The conditions necessary for measurement of the Basal Metabolic Rate are;

1. A post-absorptive state (at least 12 hours)

2. Mental and physical relaxation immediately preceding and during the test.

3. Recumbent position during the trial.

4. Awaken state

5. The environmental temperature of 20- 250°C

The factors influencing Basal Metabolism are:

A. The surface area of the person's body.

B. Age.

C. Sex.

D. Climate.

E. Racial variations.

F. The State of Nutrition.

G. Disease.

H. Effects of hormones.

The particular powerful activity of staple is the new warmth creation far beyond the caloric estimation of a given measure of nourishment, which is delivered when this nourishment is utilized by the body. There are six significant segments of the eating regimen. Sugar, fat, and protein yield vitality, accommodate development, keep up tissue exposed to mileage. Nutrients minerals and water, in spite of the fact that they don't yield energy, are a basic piece of the synthetic components for the usage of intensity and the blend of different metabolites, for example, hormones and compounds. The minerals are likewise consolidated into the structure of the tissue, and the arrangement assumes a crucial job in corrosive base equalization. Vitality for the physiologic procedure is given by the burning of sugar, fat, and protein. The everyday vitality prerequisite of day by day caloric need is the whole of the basal vitality requests in addition to that required for the extra work of the day. During periods of growth, pregnancy, or convalescence, extra calories must be provided to meet the additional demands of this process. Carbohydrate and fat "Spare" protein and thus make it available for anabolic purposes- "protein- Sparing Action" of carbohydrates and fats. This is particularly important in the nutrition of patients. The distribution of calories in the diet depends upon

A. The carbohydrate intake

B. The fat intake

C. The protein requirement and intake

D. Dietary supplements like vitamins, minerals, and water. To simplify the concept of an adequate diet for healthy individuals, foodstuffs have been arranged into four groups, each of which makes a major contribution to the diet. These groups are as follows:

1. **Milk group**: Milk, Cheese, Ice-cream, and other milk products.

2. **Meat Group**: Meat, fish, poultry eggs.

3. **Vegetables and Fruits**: Dark green or yellow vegetables, citrus fruits, or tomatoes. Some uncooked vegetables

4. **Breads and cereals**: Enriched or whole-grain breads and cereals

An eating routine that is completely helpful for the act of Yoga and profound advancement is known as the Yogic eating regimen. Diet has a private association with the psyche. The brain is shaped out of the subtlest part of nourishment. Sage Uddalaka educates his child Svetaketu "Nourishment, when devoured turns out to be triple: **the gross particles become a stool, the ordinary one's substance, and the fine ones the psyche**. My youngster, when the curd is agitated, its fine particles which rise upwards, structure margarine. In this way, my youngster, when nourishment is devoured, the fine particles which rise upwards structure the psyche. Henceforth absolutely, the brain is nourishment." Again you will discover in the Chhandogya Upanishad: "By nourishment one becomes refined in his internal nature; by the sanitization of his inward nature he verily gets a memory of the Self; and by the achievement of the memory of the Self, all ties and connections are cut off."

Diet is of three sorts viz., **Sattvic diet, Rajasic diet, and Tamasic diet**. Milk, grain, wheat, oats, spread, cheddar, tomatoes, nectar, dates, natural products, almonds, and sugar-candy are all Sattvic groceries. They render the psyche untouched and quiet. Fish, eggs, meat, salt, chilies, and asafoetida are Rajasic staples. They energize enthusiasm. Hamburger, wine, garlic, onions, and tobacco are Tamasic staples. They fill the brain with outrage, obscurity, and idleness.

Ruler Krishna says to Arjuna: "The nourishment which is of high repute to each is triple. Hear the differentiations of these. The nourishments which increment essentialness, vitality, force, wellbeing, and delight and which are flavorful, dull, significant, and pleasant are of high repute to the untouched. The enthusiastic want nourishments that are severe, sharp, saline, too much hot, impactful, dry, and consuming and which produce torment, grief, and illness. The nourishment which is stale, dull, foul and spoiled, leavings and debased is of high repute to the Tamasic."

Nourishment has a significant influence on contemplation. Various nourishments produce various impacts on multiple compartments of the mind. For purposes of reflection, the food ought to be light, nutritious, and Sattvic. Milk, organic products, almonds, spread, sugar-treats, green gram, Bengal gram absorbed water medium-term, bread, and so forth., are on the whole exceptionally accommodating in contemplation. Thed (a sort of root accessible in wealth in the Himalayan areas) is very Sattvic. Tea and sugar ought to be utilized with some restraint. It is better on the off chance that you can surrender them altogether. Dried ginger-powder can be blended in with milk and taken much of the time. Indian Yogins like this without question. Another wellbeing giving stuff is myrobalan of the yellow assortment, which can be bitten every so often. In the Vagbhata, it is spoken to as even better than a sustaining mother. It deals with the body better than a mother does. A mother gets irritated with her kid now and again, yet myrobalan consistently keeps an even personality and is merry and eager to take care of the prosperity of individuals. It jellies semen and stops every nighttime emanation. Potato, bubbled without salt or prepared ablaze, is additionally brilliant nourishment for experts.

An amateur ought to be cautious in picking the nourishment stuff of Sattvic nature. Nourishment practices enormously tremendous impact over the brain. You can see it clearly in regular day to day existence. It is hard to control mind after an overwhelming, lavish, inedible, sumptuous feast. The brain runs, meanders, and hops like a primate regularly. Liquor causes extraordinary energy at the top of the priority list.

Development is superior to the insurgency. You ought not to roll out unexpected improvements in anything, especially so in issues of nourishment and drink. Leave the change alone, moderate, and progressive. The framework ought to suit it with no difficulty—nature non-agit per saltum (nature never moves by jumps).

Nourishment is just a mass of vitality. Water and air additionally supply energy to the body. You can live without food for a few days, yet you can't live without air, in any event, for a couple of moments. Oxygen is considerably progressively significant. What is needed to take care of the body is vitality. On the off chance that you can supply this vitality by some other methods, you can completely shed nourishment. Yogins live without nourishment by drinking nectar. This nectar moves through an opening in the sense of taste. It spills and feeds the body. A Jnani can draw vitality legitimately from his unadulterated, powerful will and bolster the body with no nourishment at all. If you know the way toward bringing the vitality from the Cosmic Energy, at that point, you can keep up the body for any period and can abstain from nourishment completely.

Nourishment is of four sorts. Some liquids are drunk, solids which are pulverized by the teeth and eaten; some semi-solids are taken in by licking, and there are delicate articles that are gulped without biting. All particles of nourishment ought to be altogether chewed in the mouth until they are decreased to a significant fluid before being swallowed. At that point, no one but they can be promptly processed, retained, and acclimatized in the framework.

The eating regimen ought to be, for example, can keep up physical effectiveness and great wellbeing. The prosperity of an individual relies more upon ideal nourishment than on whatever else. Different sorts of intestinal ailments expanded defenselessness to irresistible maladies, absence of high imperativeness and intensity of obstruction, rickets, scurvy, iron deficiency, or poverty of blood, beriberi. So forth., are because of inadequate nourishment. It ought to be recollected that it can't a lot of the atmosphere as nourishment, which assumes a fundamental job in delivering a hearty and sound body or a weakling experiencing a large group of sicknesses. Apparent information on the study of dietetics is necessary for everyone, particularly for profound hopefuls, to stay aware of physical proficiency and great wellbeing. Wannabes ought to have the option to make out a modest and even eating regimen from just certain particles of nourishment. What is required is an even eating routine, not a greasy eating regimen. A rich eating routine produces sicknesses of the liver, kidneys, and pancreas. An even eating routine encourages a man to develop, to turn out more work, expands his body-weight, and keeps up the effectiveness, stamina, and an elevated requirement of buoyant energy. Your health will depend on the type of food you eat.

Indulgent people and epicureans can't fantasy about getting achievement in Yoga. He who takes a moderate eating regimen, which has directed his eating regimen can turn into a Yogi, not others. That is the motivation behind why Lord Krishna says: "Verily Yoga can't him who eateth to an extreme, nor who avoided to overabundance, nor who is a lot of dependent on rest, nor even to alertness, O Arjuna! Yoga killeth out all torment for him who is managed in eating and beguilement, controlled in performing activities, directed in dozing and waking.". Accordingly, take charming, healthy, and sweet nourishment half-stomachful; fill a quarter stomach with water and permit the rest of the quarter stomach free for extension of gas. Offer up the demonstration to the Lord. This is a moderate eating routine.

All articles that are rotten, stale, deteriorated, unclean, twice-cooked, kept medium-term, ought to be surrendered. The eating routine ought to be new, straightforward, light, tasteless, healthy, effectively edible, and nutritious. He who lives to eat is a heathen; however, he who eats to live is most likely a holy person. In the Siva Samhita, it is stated: "Yoga ought not to be drilled following a feast, nor when one is extremely eager; before starting the training, some milk and margarine ought to be taken."

You will discover in the Yoga-Tattva Upanishad: "The capable in Yoga should desert the nourishment adverse to the act of Yoga. He should surrender salt, mustard, harsh things, hot, impactful or unpleasant articles, asafoetida, ladies, squandering of the body by fasts, and so on. During the beginning times of training, nourishment of milk and ghee is appointed; additionally, nourishment comprising of wheat, green heartbeat, and red rice is said to support the advancement. At that point, he will have the option to hold his breath as long as he can imagine. By in this way, holding the breath as long as he can imagine, Kevala-Kumbhaka (suspension of breath without inward breath and exhalation) is achieved. When Kevala-Kumbhaka is achieved by one, and in this way inward breath and exhalation are abstained from, there is nothing out of reach in the three universes to him."

In the Bhikshuka-Upanishad, you will discover: "Paramahamsas like Samavartaka, Aruni, Svetaketu, Jada Bharata, Dattatreya, Suka, Vamadeva, Haritaki, and others take eight pieces and make progress toward Moksha alone through the way of Yoga."

Manu, Jesus, and Buddha encouraged the individuals to abstain from utilizing alcohol, intoxicants, and medications as these are injurious in their belongings. No otherworldly advancement is conceivable without forsaking them.

By far, most of the people burrow their graves through their teeth. No rest is given to the stomach. All things considered, man needs next to no on this abundant earth—a couple of portions of bread, a little spread, and some virus water. This will adequately do the trick to prop the life up. Individuals, unexpectedly, stuff their stomachs with a wide range of things, consumable and uneatable, because of the power of propensity in any event, when there is no hunger. This is extremely terrible. All ailments take their starting point in overburdening the stomach. Appetite is the best sauce. On the off chance that there is hunger, nourishment can be processed well. If you have no hunger, don't take anything. Let the stomach appreciate a full occasion.

An assortment of dishes exhausts the stomach, prompts eccentric hunger, and renders the tongue particular. At that point, it gets hard to satisfy the tongue. Consequently, control the tongue first; at that point, the various faculties can be effortlessly managed. Man has prepared too many kinds of dishes just to please his sense of taste and made life complicated and hopeless. When he is ignorant and fooled by the faculties, he considers himself an acculturated man. When he can't get his usual dishes in another place, his brain gets irritated. Is that real quality? He was a flat out tongue slave. This is completely disgusting. For eating and drinking, be natural and simple. Equilibrium is Meditation. Food to live, do not eat to live. Keep this quality good, and be glad. Then you might devote more time to Yoga rehearses.

A Yogic understudy who invests his energy entirely in unadulterated contemplation needs next to no nourishment. One or one and a half soothsayers of milk and a few organic products for every day will very get the job done. In any case, a Yogi who climbs the stage for fiery, dynamic work needs copious, nutritious nourishment.

A veggie lover diet has been acclaimed to be generally helpful for profound and clairvoyant headway. It has been discovered that meat enlarges creature energy and diminishes the scholarly limit. While the facts demonstrate that meat-eating nations are truly dynamic and solid, the equivalent can't be said of their profound accomplishments. Meat can't be all essential for the keeping up of flawless wellbeing, life, and essentialness. Despite what might be expected, it is exceptionally destructive to wellbeing. It acquires its train a large group of infirmities, for example, tapeworm, albuminuria, and different illnesses of the kidneys.

Meat-eating and liquor abuse are firmly unified. The longing for alcohol kicks the bucket a characteristic passing when the meat is pulled back. The topic of contraception turns out to be exceptionally troublesome on account of the individuals who take meat. To them, mind-control is alongside outlandish. Imprint how the meat-eating tiger and the dairy animals or elephant living on green grass are posts into pieces! The one is wild and fierce; the other is gentle and quiet. Meat affects the various compartments of the mind.

    The most important step in the otherworldly progression of an applicant is the surrendering of meat. The Divine Light won't plummet if the stomach is stacked with meat. In huge meat-eating nations, malignant growth mortality is exceptionally high. Veggie lovers keep up sound wellbeing till mature age. Indeed, even in the West, specialists in emergency clinics put patients on a routine of vegetable eating regimen. They convalesce rapidly. It is an inviting sign to see that at any rate in a portion of the nations of Europe, veggie lover lodgings are jumping up in astounding numbers. It can't a lot to anticipate that in 10 years or two, the Westerners will turn out to be a significant diverse race of individuals out and out in their nourishment, dress, habits, propensities, and social traditions.

Pythagoras appears to bewail when he says: "Be careful, O humans, of contaminating your bodies with corrupt nourishment. There are oats; the natural products somewhere near their weight twist their leaves, and the grapes on the vines are lush. There are sweet vegetables and herbs, which can make the fire smooth and appropriate. Neither are you denied milk, nor nectar, the scent of the blooming thyme. The fertile earth provides you with an abundance of unadulterated nourishment and accommodates practical suppers without gore and butcher.

Fasting is prohibited for experts of Yoga as it produces shortcoming. Be that as it may, intermittent mellow fasts are exceptionally useful. They will update the framework altogether, offer rest to the stomach and the digestive organs, and dispose of uric corrosive. Yogic understudies may take one full feast at 11 o'clock, some warm milk toward the beginning of the day, and a large portion of a diviner of milk and a few plantains (or oranges or apples) around evening time with numerous focal points. The night supper ought to be extremely light. If the stomach is over-burden, rest will follow, and as an excess of rest is hindering to Yogic practices, one can't make any genuine progress in the way of Yoga. In this manner, an eating regimen comprising of milk and natural products alone is a fantastic menu for all professionals.

Wannabes ought to stay away from all drugs, espresso, tea, liquor, and smoke that animate the faculties. Our faculties are contrasted with unsettled ponies, and they become wild by taking opiates. You should control them by avoiding taking drugs. We are on the whole captives of our faculties pretty much, and the faculties, this way, are the captives of opiates. In the event that you pine for flawlessness, control of the brain, and achievement in Yoga, stay away from these opiates by every single imaginable mean.

Bubble a large portion of a soothsayer of milk alongside some bubbled rice, ghee, and sugar. This is called Charu. This is amazing nourishment for Yogic specialists. This is for supper. A large portion of a diviner of milk and a few natural products will accomplish for the evening. Attempt this solution and disclose to me the advantages you have inferred in your Sadhana.

Milk ought not to be bubbled excessively. It ought to be expelled from the fire the minute the breaking point is reached. Exorbitant bubbling crushes every single nutritious standard and nutrients and renders milk unfit for utilization. Milk is a perfect nourishment for hopefuls. It is ideal nourishment without anyone else.

Organic product diet practices a great impact upon the constitution. This is a characteristic eating routine. Natural products are enormous vitality makers. Products of the soil help focus and reflection. Grain, wheat, milk, ghee, and nectar advance life span of life and increment force and stamina. Organic product juice and the water wherein sugar-candy is broken up generally excellent beverages.

TABLE SHOWING SATTVIC, RAJASIC AND TAMASIC ARTICLES OF DIET

SATTVIC	RAJASIC	TAMASIC	
Cow's milk, Sugar, Cheese, Butter, Curd, Ghee, Sweet Fruits, Apples, Bananas, Grapes, Papaya, Granates, Mangoes, Oranges, Pears, Pineapples, Guavas, Figs, Beans,	Peaches, almonds, pistachios, raisins, wheat, red rice, unpolished rice, grain, oats, dried peas, dates, sugar-sweets, green gram, bengal gram, green heartbeat, groundnut,	Fish, Eggs, Meat, Salt, Chillies, Chutney, Asafoetida, Pickles, Tamarind, Mustard, Sour things, Hot things, Tea, Coffee, Cocoa, Ovaltine, White sugar, Carrots, Turnips,	Beef, Pork, Wine, Onions, Garlic, Tobacco, Rotten things, Stale things, Unclean things, Twice cooked things, All intoxicants, All liquors, All drugs

| Coconuts, Brinjals, Carrots, Cabbages, Spinach, Tomatoes. | oats, dried ginger, myrobalan, lemon, nectar, charu. | Spices. | |

FREQUENTLY ASKED QUESTIONS

The following are questions we regularly get from tenderfoots needing to get into yoga who start with this daily practice. If you are simply beginning, you may have posed at least one of these inquiries yourself.

How long would it be advisable for you to rehearse yoga?

A decent beginning stage is focusing on three days per week simultaneously. They shouldn't be hour-long meetings you can develop as you go! Simply beginning with a 20-minute meeting (like this one) will assist you with getting results on the off chance that you are reliable.

When's the best time to rehearse this yoga schedule?

This relies upon your calendar, however, when beginning, it's a smart thought to rehearse around a similar time, particularly on the off chance that you are rehearsing yoga at home, so you start to distinguish that time as your training to assist you with building it into a propensity.

Many individuals appreciate turning out right when they get up in the first part of the day as they like to rehearse yoga on an unfilled stomach. In contrast, others appreciate rehearsing at night to enable them to loosen up. This all relies upon you and your objectives regularly if your objective is weight reduction, turning out on a vacant stomach toward the beginning of the day is best for consuming fat, however on the off chance that this can't be objective, I think whatever time causes you to appreciate the training most and return to it, over and over, is the best decision.

Would it be advisable for you to heat up before rehearsing yoga?

Indeed! Never go into a physical action without heating up. Despite the fact that this routine has a couple of represents that can be altered to make a warm-up, you need to ensure you do a couple of delicate represents that wake up your whole body to maintain a strategic distance from injury and get you in the right outlook.

Do you need rest days from yoga?

On the off chance that you feel sore in the wake of rehearsing yoga, or any kind of exercise so far as that is concerned, I believe it's keen to have a rest day, however that doesn't mean sitting on the lounge chair throughout the day-this can make you sorer from the absence of development.

More or less, you're sore from the development of lactic corrosive. To separate the lactic corrosive, you need to ensure you move and stretch; however, you would prefer not to over-stress your body. Take a stab at taking a walk or doing a loosening up yoga stream.

What do I need to begin yoga?

All you have to bring are agreeable garments and a decent mentality. We do an assortment of developments in a yoga class, so your garments ought to have the option to move unreservedly with you. A few classes may make you sweat, so dress likewise.

Imagine a scenario in which I have never done yoga.

Don't sweat it! You can see somebody in participation to talk about what you are searching for in a yoga class, and they can control you to the correct class.

Imagine a scenario where I have a physical issue or state of being.

To begin with, check with your doctor and ensure it is alright. It is likewise significant for you to register with the educator before class on the off chance that you have any worries. Yoga is NO Competition! No Comparison! We ought not to think about how we did a represent the prior week because consistently is new. Tune in to your body, and if it says to chill out, at that point, ease off! Nobody is making a decision about you; it's your body, your training.

What if I fart?

Truly, this happens a ton in yoga! At the point when you are curving, bowing, and extending, they may find you napping! If you pass gas, don't stress over it! On the off chance that you disregard it, so will every other person. Educators are utilized to it and will regularly converse with diverting their consideration. On the off chance that it is an issue for you routinely, at that point, consider being aware of what you eat before class and maintain a strategic distance from huge suppers a couple of hours before class.

Imagine a scenario in which I nod off or wheeze during Savasana.

Bravo for being so loose! Again no stresses. Your instructor will offer a tap by walking or a few words to take you back to the room! It happens to everybody!

I'm in a bad state, would I be able to, in any case, do yoga?

No doubt, yes! If you have genuine concerns, talk with your doctor before beginning a yoga practice. On the off chance that you've essentially dropped out of an activity schedule, tune in to your body and just do what you can do, attempting to your edge, not past it. Use props and tune in to the educator's directions for altering stances to make them increasingly open. After some time, you'll develop quality, stamina, equalization, and adaptability.

How frequently would it be advisable for me to rehearse for seven days?

Once more, it's your body, your training. Everything relies upon how you feel sincerely and truly. For instance, on the off chance that you had moved toward taking hot yoga and your back was harming throughout the day: that would be an opportunity to take a night off or do therapeutic yoga rather than a difficult class.

Is there an age breaking point to rehearsing yoga?

Not in any way! We have understudies that have begun in their 60's and keep up training in their 70's and 80's! In our classes, you may see an 18-year-old and a 70-year-old in a similar class. For whatever length of time that both are tuning in to their bodies and regarding their impediments, at that point, there is no restriction to your yoga practice!

What would it be advisable for me to expect when I get the opportunity to class?

• Arrive 10-15 minutes ahead of schedule. On the off chance that the class before your group is still in the meeting, if you don't mind hold up outside the studio until it is finished.

• Disconnect. Mood killer your wireless. Try not to put it on vibrate, put it on flight mode or turn it off totally.

- Take off your shoes AS SOON AS YOU ENTER the studio. We walk shoeless in the studio, and the soil is an undesirable interruption!

- Introduce yourself to the instructor and let them know whether you are new if you have any wounds or concerns.

- Put your tangle down, get your props, and take a couple of moments left before class to be still and prepare genuinely and intellectually for class. Stretch, turn, or simply lie on your back or sit on your tangle; it doesn't make a difference. It's your body, your training!; interestingly, you start the significant procedure of giving your self over totally to yoga for the following an hour!

Since the entirety of your yoga questions has been replied, it's an ideal opportunity to quit pondering about yoga, and begin doing yoga!

Five Easy Mindfulness Meditations

The upsides of contemplation are across the board – from medical advantages to the straightforward act of relating all the more serenely to the individuals around us. Like most beneficial things, reflection requires to rehearse and can be difficult work; however, that doesn't mean it's inconceivable. By finding the kind of contemplation that is directly for you, the procedure can be entirely agreeable to be sure. We prescribe attempting every one of these contemplations for 10 minutes in the first place, at that point, broadening the time continuously as you get progressively alright with the training that suits you.

MINFULNESS

WHAT: Also known as Vipassana or knowledge contemplation, mindfulness practice involves concentrating uncovered mindfulness on the object of reflection – be it the breath, physical sensations, outside sounds, or the entirety of the above mentioned.

HOW:

1. Expect an agreeable yet ready upstanding position.

2. Tenderly carry your thoughtfulness regarding the breath, and note every inward breath and exhalation – without attempting to transform anything or take in a particular manner.

3. At the point when you notice your psyche meandering (as it unquestionably will, again and again!), tenderly take your consideration back to the breath and start once more.

WHY: According to the lessons of the Buddha, applied care reflection – alongside solid focus and fitting good direct – prompts edification or freedom from affliction. As a little something extra, care contemplation has been found to bring down pressure and battle psychological well-being issues.

MANTRA

WHAT: Mantra contemplation is like care reflection, with the expansion of a reiteration of a straightforward word or expression.

HOW:

1. Pick your mantra – it could be a straightforward word like "unwind," "tranquil," or "harmony," or something progressively profound like "ohm" or "so-murmur" (old Sanskrit words signifying "nothingness" and "I am that").

2. Expect an agreeable yet ready upstanding position, and go through 30 seconds simply sitting with your eyes shut before beginning your mantra.

3. As easily and quietly as could be allowed, start rehashing your mantra to yourself (not resoundingly), again and again. There's no compelling reason to attempt to change or stop

your considerations in any capacity – simply continue murmuring the word quietly to yourself.

WHY: The reiteration of a mantra calms the breath and, because of the brain, as indicated by New Age master Deepak Chopra, bringing the meditator into the field of "unadulterated cognizance." From a fledgling's point of view, utilizing a mantra can help center and hone a psyche inclined to meander during reflection.

STROLLING

WHAT: Walking contemplation can be similarly as significant as sitting reflection, and carries solid attention to the body and physical sensations.

HOW:

1. Pick a little, level way on which to stroll to and fro, ideally close to ten paces toward every path.

2. Before you begin moving, stop for a couple of seconds and intentionally carry your regard for the body. Notice the impressions of your feet on the ground, garments on your body, and sun and wind on your skin.

3. Start strolling as gradually as you can while as yet feeling regular, keeping your consideration inside the body. At the point when the consideration floats to outside sights or contemplations (and it will!), delicately take it back to the development in the lower half of your body – the bottoms of

your feet on the ground, the bowing and reaching out of the knee and the twist of your toes.

WHY: The basic exercise of venturing from foot to foot makes a thoughtful state, quieting the psyche and developing more keen mindfulness. Strolling contemplation can be an awesome venturing stone to focusing on careful all aspects of the day – from strolling to work to cooking or doing the dishes.

REPRESENTATIONS

WHAT: Guided representations or symbolism bring the meditator into a profoundly loosened upstate, to envision a specific scene.

HOW:

1. Locate a calm territory and sit in an agreeable position.

2. Close your eyes and inhale profoundly, and start to picture yourself in a quiet domain – maybe a vacant seashore, a mountain, or even only a patio lounger.

3. Connect the entirety of your faculties by envisioning how your serene spot looks, feels, sounds, smells, and even tastes. The more strikingly you catch your envisioned area, the more prominent the recuperating impacts of the strategy, as per specialists.

4. To improve the experience, you can tune in to encompassing sounds identified with your envisioned condition (for example, a chronicle of sea waves in case you imagine a seashore). You can likewise evaluate these chronicles and contents to control you through the activity.

WHY: Guided representations have been found to bring down circulatory strain and stress hormone levels by calming the body and the brain. Explicit representations can likewise be utilized to help accomplish explicit objectives, by envisioning achievement and certainty before the occasion.

BRAINWAVE ENTRAINMENT

WHAT: Also known as soundwave contemplation or binaural beats, brainwave reflection utilizes music on five distinct frequencies - Beta, Alpha, Theta, Delta, and Gamma – to get to and adjust various degrees of the intuitive psyche.

HOW:

1. Pick the advantage you'd prefer to deal with - Alpha for innovativeness and profound unwinding; Beta for center and focus; Theta for reflection, understanding, and memory; Delta for profound rest and mending; and Gamma to expand insight and improve IQ.

2. Pick an agreeable position – either sitting or setting down – and go through a moment or two loosening up your body.

3. Play some music from the recurrence you'd prefer to chip away at (the connections above are an incredible spot to begin), and spotlight on what you want, utilizing inventive representation and positive self-converse with begin constructing new neural pathways bit by bit. Clutch that idea/picture/feeling as long as you can.

WHY: Brainwave contemplation can't unwinding - experts trust it can open your psyche to new thoughts, move you, and help you to think all the more inventively.

SIXTEEN PRINCIPLES OF SELF DEFENSE

For a considerable length of time, brutality has been a reality for ladies everywhere throughout the world. Indeed, even today, where ladies are driving multi-billion-dollar organizations, bearing duties in key government positions, winning for the family, and turning out to be specialists of progress, ladies keep on being exposed to mental and physical brutality. While the level of viciousness shifts – from wolf whistles, lustful gazes, being contacted improperly, to frightful assault, its effect doesn't.

Each time, it is an infringement of poise and an essential human right. This has prompted various discussions on how we can bring a change and make work environments, homes, urban communities, and boulevards more secure for ladies. One of these is simply the requirement for ladies to learn protection. While most recognize that it is significant, much uncertainty if such preparation would help when confronted with a real emergency, and the body and brain freeze. This is the place yoga and self-protection meet up

Terrific Master Akshar, Founder of Akshar Yoga, a well-known yoga foundation chain in Bengaluru, says, "Yoga, as craftsmanship assists train with peopling in 'determination.' One of the outcomes of rehearsing asanas is that we figure out how to hold persuasive stances and conquer the rush of feelings that emerge from them. Self-restraint and mental quality originate from such practices. What's more, these characteristics are simply the premise barrier." He includes, "A genuine yogi or yogini doesn't comprehend the idea of 'quitting any pretense of.' Commenting on this, the yoga master reasons, "To be cognizant, prepared for potential dangers, to guarantee that you are proactive and not responsive, to be engaged, certain and solid: this is the thing that yoga instructs us. This is additionally the acquired head for all your other self-preservation strategies. Yoga itself is simply the reason for all 'cutting edge' protection philosophies."

Discussing how there has been a moderate yet obvious development of why individuals rehearsed this old otherworldly craftsmanship, he says, "Yoga is every one of that was, all that is and all that is destined to be." A short delay later, he says, "In any case, the inspiration to rehearse this awesome workmanship may have changed starting with one period then onto the next. In the past, yoga was polished in mystery and private spaces; contrast that and today, you will see the situation isn't the equivalent. Presently, the method of reasoning of learning the specialty of yoga inclines more toward creating life, achieving wellbeing, and satisfaction." He clarifies further, "a definitive objective of yoga is harmony. In any case, in the present reality, it is trying to accomplish harmony without having achieved quality. Keeping that in mind, yoga and self-protection are commonly comprehensive and associated."

LADIES, YOGA, AND SELF-DEFENSE: HOW THE SPECKS ASSOCIATE

"Yoga stirs what we call, Shakti vitality. Furthermore, through yoga and reflection, ladies can connect with themselves and understand their actual worth and potential. The entire idea of 'men are more grounded' is settled. Through yoga, ladies build up the current certainty to coordinate with their partners as equivalents," says Akshar. A motivation behind why yoga in self-preservation varies from different systems is that "the guideline of yogic self-protection is self-acknowledgment and securing this self." While it sounds enabling, the inquiry presented by numerous who connect ladies' capacities and qualities with their age – can ladies of any age learn yoga in self-preservation? Akshar says, "Ladies from varying backgrounds can procure and even ace this ability. The proverb 'age is only a number' is valid here." another development in self-preservation Akshar accepts that the three most significant variables with regards to self-protection for ladies are: fitness, certainty, and awareness. These likewise correspond with the quest for a yogi.

The principles of self-defense include:

1. **Extravagant moves and confused movements have no spot in any self-protection preparation.**

The more perplexing the activity, the almost certain it is to self-destruct when confronted with the pressure of a genuine self-preservation squabble. Or maybe, preparing should concentrate on basic and essential developments that set aside little effort to execute and are less inclined to "administrator blunders." So on the off chance that you are being shown flying armbars and turning hopping back kicks as a significant staple of your self-protection preparing, you most likely ought to reevaluate your preparation.

On a side note, simplicity of execution doesn't imply that the understudy ought to hope to put a brief period into their preparation. Indeed, even the straightforward things set aside some effort to consummate and expect the practice to strengthen and sharpen in the abilities. So consistent practice is as yet required.

2. Quicker is better

This standard identifies with the past point. Less difficult moves should take less time to execute than perplexing movements. In a self-preservation situation, the outlook ought to be to shield and quickly assault the assailant. The quicker we hurt them, the less they hurt us. Parts of a second issue in a desperate battle, so mind-boggling entries that expect longer to execute ought to be energized less in preparing then clear punches, kicks, knees, elbows, hammer clench hands, and different strikes to helpless focuses on that promptly dispense harm to the assailant.

3. Plan for the obscure

A definitive objective is to expect the unforeseen. Or, on the other hand, even better, the preparation should represent the unforeseen. Given that we can't represent all vulnerabilities, there are a couple of fundamental stipulations the preparation should contemplate to best get ready understudies to manage the obscure.

Given that an assault may happen when you wouldn't dare to hope anymore ought to be instructed to work from any position: sitting, lying, remaining, in limited spaces, and so forth.

4. Understudies ought to consistently be educated to examine different risks toward the finish of any method to abstain from being trapped by another assailant.

Dependence on quality alone ought to be debilitated when preparing to safeguard yourself. The presumption should be made that the aggressor can be more grounded or greater than you, and attempting to muscle your approach to security forcefully can cause more mischief than anything. In this manner, understudies ought to be instructed to make points while guarding, also called clearing the channel, to be least presented to consequent assaults, shrouded weapons, and other potential perils.

Preparing ought to dishearten understudies from taking the battle superfluously to the ground. Development on the ground is very restricted, which incredibly lessens any odds of effectively getting away, in addition to it makes you a simpler objective for numerous aggressors and makes you progressively presented to assaults with different weapons. Preparing ought to incorporate shielding against numerous aggressors. In spite of the fact that the odds of effectively warding off various rivals are, for the most part, lower than battling a solitary individual, the preparation needs to incorporate these situations to improve the chances of achievement.

5. Methodical preparation is superior to an assortment of an immense measure of disconnected procedures.

Procedures are a beginning stage for learning self-protection. However, a genuine self-protection control ought to be a framework interconnected and associated standards and developments that, whenever educated accurately, expand upon one another. This deliberate preparation of self-preservation permits understudies the capacity to see better and disguise the strategies and the subtleties behind them instead of just depending on repetition remembrance, which can self-destruct under states of extreme pressure.

6. Stress preparing and competing is an unquestionable requirement.

Nothing in a genuine battle ever goes as easily as arranged. Consequently, preparing ought to incorporate components of managing and conquering strife, exhaustion, dread, and different snags that block the understudy's capacity to play out a strategy effectively.

7. Understudies ought to be helped that legitimate execution to remember strategy can't extreme objective in any self-protection preparing, rather it is an effective break from hurt.

The strategy is just an entryway to arriving at that objective. If the underlying strategy was fruitless or a mix-up was made in its execution, understudies must be instructed to abstain from freezing or halting and keep battling until they have effectively protected themselves and gotten away varying.

Since battling is critical to beating deterrents, striking and competing must be a customary part of any self-protection preparing to get understudies acclimated with contact and to battle.

8. Maintain a strategic distance from the battle whenever the situation allows

This rule is regularly disregarded in preparing. Be that as it may, regularly, the ideal approach to stay away from injury is to forestall strife in any case. Obviously, not generally is it conceivable to flee or leave a showdown in particular. Yet, de-heightening estimates must be instructed to understudies, and understudies ought to be urged to utilize their best judgment regarding when to battle and when to not. For instance, protections against weapon dangers ought to be instructed related to consistency with the aggressor's requests, at whatever point the assailant is requesting things of fiscal esteem and can be effectively left behind without enduring real damage all the while.

9. Convey objects equipped for making a commotion

Mobile phones, whistles, horns, and so on, anything that can make individuals aware of your circumstance. The sound from a crisis whistle can travel more remote and is more potent than just shouting for help. Self-preservation associations, for example, Safety and Self Defense Solutions likewise energize potential casualties of assaults to holler 'fire' to draw consideration and alarm off an assailant. Individuals are bound to react to somebody shouting 'fire' than to somebody hollering 'help.'

10. **Continuously recognize what devices you need to safeguard yourself and make them reachable before they are required.**

For instance, keeping your keys in your grasp while strolling to your vehicle and letting the point extend between your knuckles can be utilized as an unexpected weapon, or a monkey clench hand produced using paracord can be utilized as a viable instrument to daze an aggressor.

11. **Know your way.**

Be acquainted with the courses and ways you bring home or to your bug-out area. Realizing your way implies realizing the spots individuals could cover up and giving those zones a wide billet when passing. It likewise implies maintaining a strategic distance from dim or new alternate routes that may get you lost or cornered.

12. **Ensure somebody knows where you are and when to anticipate you.**

This is valid for some circumstances you may end up in, such as climbing, heading out to or from work, or clearing during a crisis. Keeping a dear companion or crisis contacts forward-thinking on your area is as basic as a speedy call or instant message.

13. **Walk unquestionably.**

Numerous predators are searching for somebody they want to overwhelm, much like a predator in nature. Stroll with reason and course, focusing as you go, so you keep away from shocks.

14. **Trust your senses.**

On the off chance that you figure somebody may be tailing you or are frightened by somebody close by, it's smarter to get to a bustling territory and contact somebody you trust to get you.

15. **Stay away from schedules that could without much of a stretch be followed.**

On the off chance that conceivable, abstain from doing certain exercises, such as pulling back cash or taking similar courses home, simultaneously every day.

16. **Know the delicate regions of your assailant and how these regions can be misused.**

The eyes, ears, throat, crotch, knees, and shins are on the whole territories that hurt when hit. For instance, an ear slap or crotch assault can give you the advantage.

17. **Build up a hostile attitude**.

Think regarding assaulting the aggressor, instead of safeguarding against his assault.

18. **Trust Your Instincts.**

Figure out how to tune in to your "inward voice" Let your hunch and impulse caution you of threats and notice there notice.

SURVIVAL FITNESS PLAN YOGA ROUTINE QUICK-LIST

Survival Fitness is self-preparing in the five most helpful exercises for getting away from the threat.

Show yourself parkour, climbing, swimming, riding, and climbing. It likewise has a basic day by day schedule to keep your brain and body in ideal wellbeing with negligible exertion.

Begin preparing in Survival Fitness today, since you'll get fit while learning life-sparing aptitudes!

Get it now.

Everybody Knows You Need to Exercise to Stay Healthy

Stay in shape and get life-sparing abilities simultaneously.

100% bodyweight works out

Give yourself the most obvious opportunity to get away from dangerous circumstances.

Receive all the general rewards of good wellbeing

Never get exhausted from "the regular old daily practice."

Get a good deal on exercise center charges, fitness coaches, and costly hardware.

Join the Survival Fitness Revolution

Here is a sample of what's remembered for Survival Fitness:

Parkour

Wellbeing preparing

Molding

Parity preparing

Running and bouncing abilities.

Vaulting over items

Moving over dividers

Arranging bar hindrances

Parkour games

Climbing

Key climbing standards

Holds and grasps

Foot methods

Break climbing

Swimming

METHODS AND DRILLS TO IMPROVE YOUR SWIMMING VELOCITY

Swimming ultra-long separation an endurance circumstance

The most effective method to do an extremely productive stroke created by the US Navy Seals

A full preparing guide for how to do a 50-meter submerged swim

Fundamental water salvage abilities

Riding

Crucial riding abilities

Essential and propelled riding drills.

Strategies for tough and downhill riding

Arranging impediments securely

Climbing

General climbing tips

Climbing with a pack

Explicit climbing strategies for various landscapes and climate

Every day Health and Fitness.

Straightforward breathing activities to build your imperativeness

The main two molding practices you have to keep your body agile and solid.

A 15-minute full-body yoga routine for adaptability and quality

The simplest contemplation strategy for a reasonable and quiet brain

How to do the Survival Fitness Plan Super Burpee. A warm-up, stretch, and conditioning workout all in one exercise

Burpees could be one of the hardest, most extreme pieces of an exercise meeting. This perspiration initiating, touchy four-advance development includes hunching down, pushing, getting into a board position, and hopping. "A burpee is a full-body practice that creates muscle quality and consume calories," says Kamal Chhikara, proprietor and lead trainer of the Reebok CrossFit Robust exercise center in Delhi. It connects all the significant muscle bunches like the arms, chest, quads, glutes, hamstrings, and abs.

That is maybe why it was received by the US armed force during World War II to survey the wellness levels of enlisted people and has gotten a most loved with coaches everywhere throughout the world, says Mumbai-based Shruti Kadam, wellness master at Gold's Gym, India. "Indeed, even a couple of moments of burpees increment strong continuance and coordination."

The following are the extra advantages. In any case, do recollect, in case you're new to practice when all is said in done or 40 or more in age, don't begin burpees without a coach—you could get harmed.

Useful for weight reduction

The way to fat misfortune is keeping the pulse high long enough to consume put away fat, says Vesna Pericevic Jacob, a wellness master and author of wellness focus Vesna's Alta Celo in Delhi. The burpee requests everything that is in you and force, using the muscles from your feet to the neck and shoulders.

That is not all. Your body works at busting fat in any event, when you're finished with burpees. Burpees support your digestion, so you consume more calories for the day, proposing that you finish your exercises with 3 minutes of burpees (pursue 30 redundancies) for extra weight reduction. In the middle of the road level, focus on 100-150 burpees as quickly as would be prudent, she proposes. You can add a press-up to the fundamental burpee to challenge your chest area quality.

As referenced, burpees connect most muscle gatherings; in particular, the center. A more grounded center method an actuated focal sensory system, which thus makes you alert, improves memory and body usefulness.

Make it touchy

Burpees are both unpredictable and anaerobic, intended to keep you exhausted, so the shorter and quicker the exercise, the better. For a novice, 7 minutes of burpees are sufficient, while at a propelled arrange, an insignificant 5 minutes (since you're doing burpees quicker at a propelled organize; you may do 40 burpees in a short time, versus 20 out of 10 minutes when you are an amateur) attempts to give your body an exercise.

Shock your body

Doing one exercise gets your body accustomed to it, lessening its effect. With burpees, you can test and incorporate varieties, making each exercise a shock to your body. Attempt a container hop burpee, where you bounce on to a crate before you post board as opposed to straight up and back. Different varieties incorporate bounce over burpees, where you hop over an impediment between two burpees, and fold hop burpees, where you overlap your knees into your chest at the pinnacle of the hop.

Increment of perseverance

Different redundancies of burpees, which is how it should be done, grow your lungs, making you short of breath, and make your heart more grounded, making the body used to bear more. Your body gets more grounded, prepared to confront all the more testing exercise systems; your presentation in different exercises, such as cycling, swimming, and trekking, improves as well.

Assemble muscle quality

There isn't an excessive number of activities that can construct quality speedier than burpees. Dissimilar to disconnection practices like bicep twists and tricep payoffs, burpees are a full-body workout. The assortment of developments included and muscles worked implies the advantages of burpees will be clear in your day by day life, as each physical test turns out to be only that little simpler to win. For building add-on quality for your lower body, including a wide seize the finish of an ordinary burpee.

No space issue

You needn't bother with a lot of room for burpees. You can do it at home, in the garden or even in a lodging. The main gym equipment is your own body. For a total exercise, a 15-to 20-minute meeting of three-four sets, rehashing 10-15 burpees in each set.

Add them to any exercise.

Burpees are dynamic and versatile, making them an ideal expansion to any exercise, regardless of whether you're doing a HIIT (High-Intensity Interval Training)- style or need a fast Tabata exercise whenever of the day. Burpees can be consolidated into high-intensity exercise, used to heat up before different activities, or done again and again to go about as your whole exercise. One can fuse burpees as a significant aspect of the preparation, consolidating it with any vigorous activity like cycling, running, or swimming. You can likewise add them to use training or cross-fit preparation.

Things to recollect before doing burpees

■ Make sure you can perform 10-15 great push-ups or have four a month and a half of rec center understanding to keep away from wounds because of the absence of solidarity.

- General warm-up is an absolute necessity.

- Take master guidance if you have any ailment or injury, particularly of the back, knees, or shoulders.

CONCLUSION

Though the interest for Yoga Vidya in the west is growing day by day and more and more people are turning towards yoga; this is not the same in other regions of the world. Lack of proper infrastructure and the absence of an appropriate systematized approach in the propagation of yoga are still drawbacks for broader implementation. The youngsters are being drawn away from the tradition and culture and blindly ape the hedonistic lifestyle from the western movies.

Yoga practice influences change in the way of thinking. Therefore, it is crucial to give the youth proper and systematic training in yoga.

The aims of human existence are not health and happiness, but Samadhi (unity). Preoccupation with the search for happiness and health makes us forget the essential question: what is the sense of our existence. Yoga is the best way for us to regain our birthrights and attain the goal of our human existence – and health and happiness then become natural fruits of that achievement.

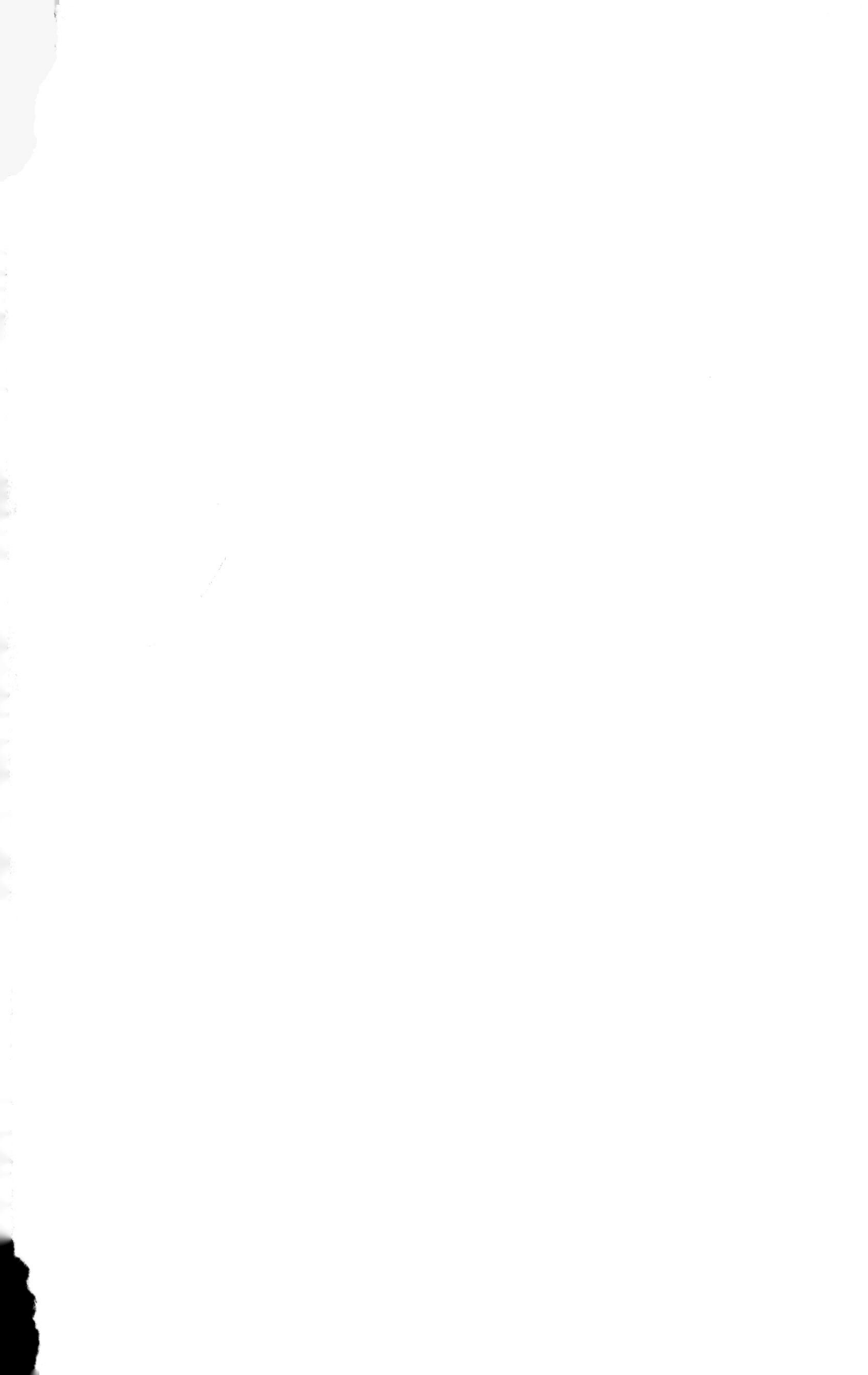

CPSIA information can be obtained
at www.ICGtesting.com
Printed in the USA
LVHW051432271120
672814LV00016B/568